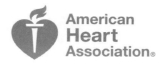

American
Heart
Association®

quick
& easy
cookbook
2ND EDITION

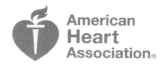

American
Heart
Association®

quick
& easy
cookbook
2ND EDITION

More Than 200 Healthy Recipes
You Can Make in Minutes

Clarkson Potter/Publishers
New York

A previous edition of this work was published in hardcover in the United
States by Times Books, New York, in 1995, and was subsequently published
in paperback by Times Books in 1998 and Clarkson Potter/Publishers, an
imprint of the Crown Publishing Group, a division of Random House, Inc.,
New York, in 2001.

Library of Congress Cataloging-in-Publication Data
Quick & easy cookbook / American Heart Association. — 2nd ed.
    p.   cm.
  Includes index.
  1. Heart—Diseases—Diet therapy—Recipes.   2. Heart—Diseases—
Prevention.   3. Low-fat diet—Recipes.   4. Low-cholesterol diet—Recipes.
I. American Heart Association.   II. Title: Quick and easy cookbook.
RC684.D5Q54   2012
641.5'6311—dc23   2011023671

ISBN 978-0-307-40761-0
eISBN 978-0-307-95387-2

Printed in the United States of America

Book design by Ashley Tucker
Jacket design by Rae Ann Spitzenberger
Jacket photography by Ben Fink

10   9   8

Second Edition

contents

acknowledgments

American Heart Association Consumer Publications
DIRECTOR: Linda S. Ball
MANAGING EDITOR: Deborah A. Renza
SENIOR EDITOR: Janice Roth Moss
SCIENCE EDITOR/WRITER: Jacqueline Fornerod Haigney
ASSISTANT EDITOR: Roberta Westcott Sullivan

Recipe Developers
Ellen Boeke
Nancy S. Hughes
Annie King
Jackie Mills, M.S., R.D.
Julie Shapero, R.D., L.D.
Linda Foley Woodrum

Nutrition Analyst
Tammi Hancock, R.D.

preface

The American Heart Association continues to be committed to bringing you sound advice on how to eat for good health and cook for good flavor. In this second edition of the *American Heart Association Quick & Easy Cookbook*, one of our first and most popular cookbooks, we also focus on showing you how to spend less time in the kitchen but still get great results at the table. This latest edition has been updated for today's modern family. It includes more than 60 new recipes that reflect current tastes, trends, and techniques, as well as the influences of diverse cuisines from around the world. Just as important, the recipes and dietary information in this new edition are based on practical and scientifically sound recommendations that come from leading experts on good nutrition.

Most of us face juggling the demands of work and family while still finding ways to eat a healthy diet. If you sometimes wonder whether it's worth the time and effort to cook at home or read labels when you shop, let me assure you that it is. Research from the nutrition community continues to demonstrate that the foods we choose every day do indeed have an important effect on our health. We at the American Heart Association have made it our business to show you how to make the most of your time in the kitchen and grocery store so you can eat well and live a heart-smart lifestyle. Now it's time for you, with the help of this cookbook, to take charge of your health—one delicious meal at a time.

Rose Marie Robertson, M.D.
CHIEF SCIENCE OFFICER
AMERICAN HEART ASSOCIATION/AMERICAN STROKE ASSOCIATION

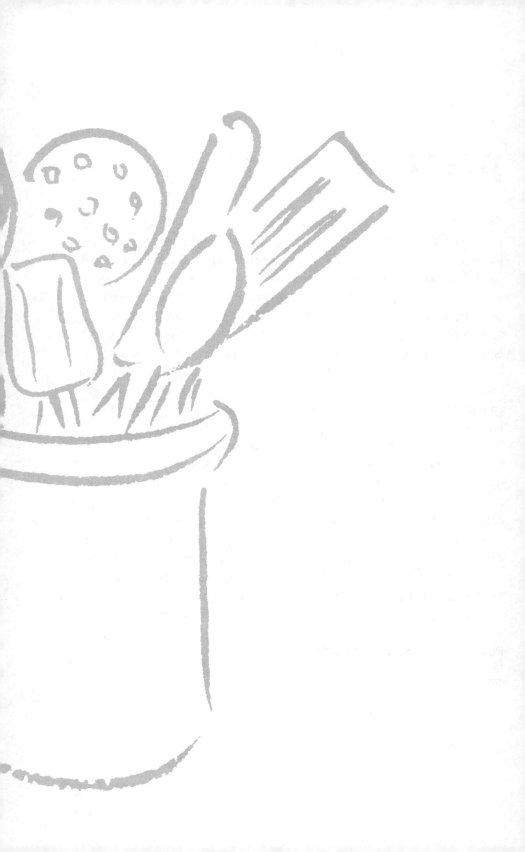

quick & easy 1·2·3

No matter how busy life gets, one constant remains: We all need to eat. Over the past few decades, however, the ways we meet that basic need have changed dramatically. With today's hectic lifestyles, it's tempting to opt out of cooking altogether, especially now that fast food is available on almost every corner. Yet taking a convenient shortcut instead of preparing meals at home can also shortchange your health. If you're looking for a better alternative to takeout and convenience foods, cooking healthy meals at home is the smartest way to go—and putting those healthy meals on the table doesn't have to take any more time than you're spending now to get processed foods.

Delicious, wholesome food needn't depend on elaborate recipes or complicated cooking techniques; all you need are a bit of forethought and a handful of nutritious ingredients. This cookbook can't add hours to your day, but it *can* offer you some simple techniques and quick and easy recipes so you can make the most of your time and enjoy meals that are both fast and flavorful.

When we say "quick and easy," we mean it. For all the recipes in this book, we have pared down the preparation time—everything you do before the cooking begins—to 20 minutes or less. In many cases, you should be able to put a meal on the table in about 30 minutes or less. (We've estimated how long both prep and cooking will take for every recipe so you'll know what to expect.) Among the quickest recipes, you'll find classic favorites such as Crunchy Fish Nuggets with Lemon Tartar Sauce (page 76) and intriguing new selections such as Jerked Salmon with Raspberry-Mint Salsa (page 80), both ready in just minutes.

It's one thing for a meal to be quick, but it's another matter to provide both quality nutrition and taste—and this book delivers on all counts. Because our recipes are developed according to the American Heart Association's dietary recommendations, you can trust that each dish will be nutritious and full of flavor. We know that a recipe isn't worth making if it isn't worth eating, so you can be sure that each recipe in this book is as delicious as it is quick to prepare.

This cookbook also offers practical strategies and tips to make choosing and preparing food as easy as 1–2–3. You'll find detailed sections that show you how to:

1. Create weekly meal plans that work with your lifestyle to provide good nutrition.
2. Make smarter choices and spend less time in the grocery store.
3. Organize your kitchen and equipment and use cooking techniques that will help get things done fast and without fuss.

Mastering the basics of good planning, smart shopping, and kitchen efficiency will make cooking at home a rewarding experience, not a chore. Everything you need to create fast and flavorful meals—tonight and every night—is right here in the second edition of the *American Heart Association Quick & Easy Cookbook.*

1 · planning principles

When time is limited, it pays to plan ahead. Following some basic meal-planning strategies will help you maximize the nutritional value of the food you cook at home while minimizing the time you spend in the kitchen.

PLAN ON PAPER

Everyone has obligations and time limitations they must work around in the course of daily life. Using a written chart will make it easier for you to keep track of when you'll have time to cook, which favorite dishes will fit into your schedule, and what to add to your grocery list.

First, identify your established eating habits and make them part of your menu plans. If you're like most people, you've developed a certain routine for breakfast and lunch that's repeated throughout the week. Pencil in those "givens" on a simple chart with columns for every day of the week. While you're at it, look for ways to increase the nutritional value of those go-to foods. For example, if you and your children eat cereal every morning, choose whole-grain varieties, switch to fat-free milk, and add fresh fruit.

Next, focus on planning your dinners to complement your breakfast and lunch standbys and build in both variety and balanced nutrition. To simplify and speed things up, you can develop a pattern of dinner entrées. The Quick & Easy Weekly Dinner Planner on page 4 is intended as a starting place to give you ideas. You'll see that the planner covers one week of dinners, with an abbreviated shopping list built in so that once you've done your planning, you'll be ready to grab your list and go. (You'll find a blank template in Appendix A that you can copy and use in your planning.) Our sample plan is based on the following pattern, but you can choose any entrée types you like, mixing and matching to suit your needs. We do, however, suggest serving fish at least twice a week and including at least one vegetarian dinner weekly.

- MONDAY — vegetarian entrée
- TUESDAY — fish entrée
- WEDNESDAY — poultry entrée
- THURSDAY — meat entrée
- FRIDAY — leftover or freezer night
- SATURDAY — fish entrée
- SUNDAY — meat or poultry entrée

QUICK & EASY WEEKLY DINNER PLANNER

	dinner menu plan	fresh/frozen ingredients	pantry staples
MON	Tangy Yogurt-Tomato Fusilli (page 176) with Mixed green salad	6 oz fat-free plain Greek yogurt Lemon zest 1 cup frozen edamame Salad ingredients	8 oz whole-grain fusilli 1 14.5-oz can no-salt-added diced tomatoes Check for garlic, rosemary, and capers
TUES	Creole Catfish (page 74) with Broccoli Instant brown rice	2 8-oz catfish fillets ½ rib celery ¼ red bell pepper ¼ onion Broccoli	1 14.5-oz can no-salt-added diced tomatoes Instant brown rice Check for garlic, paprika, and cayenne
WED	Light Chicken Chili* (page 119) with Mixed green salad *Can double recipe to freeze	1 lb boneless chicken breasts 1 onion Salad ingredients	2 cups fat-free, low-sodium chicken broth 1 4-oz can green chiles 2 15.5-oz cans no-salt-added navy beans Check for garlic and cumin
THURS	Sirloin with Orange-Coriander Glaze (page 148) with Red potatoes Asparagus	1 lb boneless top sirloin ¼ cup frozen orange juice concentrate Red potatoes Asparagus	Check for coriander, garlic powder, and cayenne
FRI	Leftover or freezer night (for example, Light Chicken Chili from Wednesday)		
SAT	Spinach-Topped Salmon (page 81) with Colorful Lemon Couscous (page 213)	4 4-oz salmon fillets 2 green onions 5 oz frozen chopped spinach ¼ cup shredded low-fat mozzarella 2 lemons 1 green and 1 red bell pepper	½ cup dry white wine 1 cup fat-free, low-sodium chicken broth 1 cup uncooked whole-wheat couscous Check for nutmeg, bay leaf, and garlic
SUN	Chicken with Leeks and Tomatoes (page 111) with Toasted Barley Pilaf (page 208)	1 lb boneless chicken breast halves 1 leek 1 cup cherry tomatoes Celery	2¼ cups fat-free, low-sodium chicken broth 1 cup uncooked pearl barley Check for sage and rosemary

PLAN TO MAXIMIZE NUTRITIOUS FOODS

Your first goal when you start meal planning is to find a combination of nutritious foods that works for you and your family. Aim for a daily balance of the primary food groups discussed below, distributing the servings across the week in any way you like. The idea is to choose a wide variety of foods so you'll get the full spectrum of nutritional benefits. You should also cut back on foods that are low in nutrition but high in calories. In your planning, tailor the number of servings from each food group to meet your individual calorie needs. On pages 259 and 260, you'll find a chart of suggested servings for each food group for different calorie levels, along with some examples of serving sizes for several common foods.

Once you find a pattern that you like, work it! Remember that you can repeat the basic elements while endlessly varying your choices from each food group. In general, make nutritious foods your go-to choices as you plan your weekly menus.

Vegetables and fruits are essential sources of vitamins, minerals, and fiber. Because they're also low in calories, these foods can help you manage your weight; a diet rich in the nutrients and minerals found in vegetables and fruits can also help lower your blood pressure. Take advantage of many different kinds of produce; the broader the variety of items you eat, the broader the range of nutrients you'll get. Incorporate different vegetables and fruits into your weekly plan, and experiment with ones you haven't tried before to find new flavors and textures you like. Deeply colored varieties are generally the most nutritious.

QUICK PICKS Red—bell peppers, beets, tomatoes, and strawberries; blue—blueberries and eggplant; green—bell peppers, beans, spinach, broccoli, and dark lettuces; orange—carrots, sweet potatoes, cantaloupe, and oranges; and yellow—summer squash.

Fat-free and low-fat dairy products are an important part of a well-rounded diet and provide calcium and protein without the saturated fat, cholesterol, and calories of whole milk and other whole-fat dairy products. Try to minimize your intake of whole-fat products. If you don't find fat-free options, look for 1 percent milk and other low-fat dairy products.

QUICK PICKS Fat-free, 1 percent, and low-fat versions of milk, half-and-half, yogurt, cheeses (lowest sodium available), sour cream, ricotta, and ice cream.

Fiber-rich whole grains provide more nutrients than processed grains, which have had the kernel and bran removed. For the most health benefits, try to use whole grains for at least half your daily servings of grain. Their fiber can work to lower your blood cholesterol and help you feel full, which can make it easier to reach and maintain a healthy weight.

> **QUICK PICKS** Whole grains (brown rice, bulgur, barley, and quinoa), whole-wheat and other whole-grain breads and rolls (lowest sodium available), whole-grain pastas (spaghetti, rotini, linguine, macaroni, penne, and others), and oatmeal and other whole-grain cereals (lowest sodium available).

Fish, especially those varieties rich in omega-3 fatty acids, should be a regular part of your weekly diet. In fact, eating these types of fish may help reduce the risk of death from coronary heart disease. The American Heart Association recommends that you eat at least two servings of fish (3 to 3½ ounces cooked, or about 4 ounces raw) each week. Try different types of seafood and preparation techniques for variety. (Children, pregnant women, and those concerned about mercury should avoid fish with the highest potential of mercury contamination, such as shark, swordfish, tilefish, and mackerel. Remember, however, that for most people, the benefits far outweigh the risks.) Most fish and shellfish are high in protein and low in saturated fat, but be aware that some shellfish, such as shrimp, are high in cholesterol.

> **QUICK PICKS** Salmon, tuna, trout, herring, and other fish rich in omega-3 fatty acids.

Lean and extra-lean meats and poultry provide protein and other important nutrients. Depending on your daily calorie needs, though, it's best to eat no more than about 6 ounces of cooked lean, low-saturated-fat poultry or meat (8 ounces before cooking) each day. When planning to use poultry, remember that the white meat is leaner than the dark and that you should discard the skin before eating.

> **QUICK PICKS** Beef—sirloin, round steak, flank steak, tenderloin, and 95 percent lean ground; pork—tenderloin and loin chops; poultry (skinless)—chicken breast and tenders, turkey breast and tenderloin.

Legumes, nuts, and seeds round out a balanced diet. Legumes provide both protein and fiber, making them a great substitute for meat. Use these nutritional powerhouses as the basis for at least one, if not more, vegetarian meals each week. Also include small amounts of unsalted nuts and seeds in your planning. They are rich in nutrients and provide heart-healthy unsaturated oils, but remember that they are also high in calories.

QUICK PICKS **Legumes—dried beans and lentils, peas, unsalted peanuts and peanut butter, and edamame (green soybeans); unsalted nuts and seeds—almonds, walnuts, pecans, hazelnuts (filberts), and pumpkin seeds.**

Unsaturated oils and fats provide monounsaturated and polyunsaturated fats, both of which have heart-health benefits. Vegetable oil products contain both mono- and polyunsaturated fats in varying percentages, as do nuts and seeds. The more often you can replace the unhealthy saturated fat found in products such as butter with these helpful unsaturated fats, the better.

QUICK PICKS **Canola, olive, corn, soybean, safflower, sunflower, walnut, and peanut oils. Cooking sprays deliver a fine mist of oil, which can greatly reduce the amount needed for cooking.**

SAMPLE PATTERN OF DAILY FOOD SERVINGS FOR A 2,000-CALORIE DIET

BREAKFAST	1 grain, 1 dairy, 1 fruit, 1 fat
SNACK	1 dairy, 1 fruit
LUNCH	1 protein, 2 grain, 2 vegetable
SNACK	1 dairy, 1 grain, 1 fruit
DINNER	1 protein, 2 grain, 2 vegetable, 1 fruit, 1 fat

For a person who needs about 2,000 calories a day, aim to include 4 to 5 vegetable servings, 4 to 5 fruit servings, 6 to 8 grain servings, 2 to 3 dairy servings, 2 protein servings, and 2 to 3 fat servings each day. Include 4 to 5 servings of unsalted nuts, seeds, and legumes per week.

PLAN TO MINIMIZE NUTRIENT-POOR FOODS

In addition to knowing which foods to focus on, it's important to avoid the foods that undermine good health. Sodium, saturated fat, trans fat, and dietary cholesterol are known to increase the risk of heart disease. (For more information on how these dietary choices can affect your heart, go to www.heart.org.) It's surprising how many common foods contain an unhealthy amount of one or more of these elements, so be proactive and know what's in the food you eat. (Certain cuts of meat are much lower in saturated fat and cholesterol than others, for example.) To be prepared to make good choices in the store and in restaurants, know where to find these dietary "villains" and familiarize yourself with better options.

Sodium, a major component of salt, is so prevalent in our current food supply that most people eat much more than the recommended maximum of 1,500 milligrams a day. Cut down on sodium by buying unprocessed foods and no-salt-added or low-sodium products, and find out as much as you can about the sodium levels in your favorite restaurant dishes so you can make heart-smart choices.

Added sugars offer no nutritional benefit but supply lots of calories— and therefore may challenge your efforts to maintain a healthy weight. If sugar-sweetened beverages, sugary snack foods, and sweet desserts are a large part of your daily diet, you may not be eating enough other, more nutritious foods. Read ingredient lists when you shop. If corn syrup, concentrated fruit juice, evaporated cane juice, honey, sucrose, fructose, dextrose, or any of the other telltale "-ose" sugars are among the first four ingredients listed, you are buying a high-sugar product. On average, you should limit sugar-sweetened beverages to no more than 450 calories or 36 ounces per week. (If you need fewer than 2,000 calories per day, avoid these beverages altogether.)

Saturated fat is found primarily in foods from animals, such as meats, poultry, and whole-fat dairy products, or in the tropical oils (most commonly, coconut, palm, and palm kernel) that are used in commercially prepared foods. Eating too much saturated fat can increase the level of harmful LDL cholesterol in your blood, which in turn increases your risk of heart disease. The easiest ways to cut down on saturated fat are to eat no more than 6 ounces of cooked lean meat or poultry each day, include vegetarian meals in your diet, and replace full-fat dairy products with fat-free or low-fat versions.

Trans fat, or trans fatty acids, results from the process of adding hydrogen to liquid vegetable oils to make them more solid. Many food manufacturers traditionally have used these partially hydrogenated oils in fried and baked products, but because we now know that a regular diet high in trans fat will increase your risk of heart disease, many products have been reformulated. Be sure to compare labels when you're choosing snack products, cakes, cookies, pastries, pies, muffins, and fried foods.

Cholesterol that is present in food comes exclusively from animal sources (meat, poultry, shellfish, and dairy products). A cholesterol-rich diet may contribute to higher levels of blood cholesterol, so it makes sense to keep your dietary cholesterol low, especially if you already have heart disease or high blood cholesterol. Certain foods, such as egg yolks, shrimp and several other shellfish, organ meats such as liver, and whole milk, are especially high in cholesterol. Try to keep track of how much cholesterol you eat each day and adjust your food choices accordingly. If you eat a three-egg omelet for breakfast, for example, cut back on other high-cholesterol items for a few days to compensate.

PLAN FOR EFFICIENCY

Using some simple time-saving strategies can really make your planning quicker and easier. Set a specific time to plan each week—and stick to it. When you begin, look through the fridge, freezer, and pantry to see what you might be able to use in the next few days. For example, refrigerated pasta is great in a casserole, and leftover roast chicken can be the base of a delicious soup or salad. Then choose a few recipes that look interesting, and put the ingredients you'll need to buy on your shopping list. Add an unfamiliar food to your plan once in a while—experimenting with new things will keep your meals interesting.

The following ideas can help you prepare meals more efficiently. (Refer to Appendix C for some helpful food-safety tips for leftovers.)

PLAN TO COOK WHEN YOU HAVE THE MOST TIME

- Plan for success. Be realistic about what is reasonable to do in the time you have. Your planning will be helpful only if it works for you and your family.

- Choose simpler recipes with fewer ingredients and fewer steps when you are the busiest. Prepare meals that need more prep on weekends or whenever your schedule allows.

- Do as much prep work as you can for your week's menu ahead of time.

COOK FAVORITE STAPLES IN LARGE QUANTITIES

- Make extra brown rice to keep on hand in either the refrigerator or the freezer. On a busy night, microwave it, stirring occasionally, until heated through, then use as you would fresh.

- Plan for two pasta meals in a week: Cook one night and boil twice as much as you need. Use the extra as the base for a later dish, or include it in soups and salads.

- Cook more couscous than you need for one meal; it reheats very well and makes a great addition to salads.

- Clean, prep, and cook more vegetables than you need for one meal. You'll have them on hand to throw into an omelet, a soup, a casserole, or a pasta dish—or just reheat, sprinkle with herbs, and serve.

DOUBLE UP ON THE MEATS AND POULTRY YOU USE

- If you know you'll be browning ground meat for one recipe in your plan, buy extra. Brown it all, but refrigerate or freeze the extra to use for a second meal later in the week.

- Baking, poaching, grilling, or broiling chicken breasts is easy and quick; save even more time by cooking twice as many pieces as you need right away. Use the extra chicken in an entrée salad, in soup, or as the base for a quickly made entrée on another day.

INCLUDE AT LEAST ONE DOUBLE-DUTY ENTRÉE EACH WEEK

- Choose at least one recipe that will provide two nights' worth of meals. When you cook casseroles, stews, and soups, make larger quantities than you need for one meal and refrigerate or freeze the extra for an encore a few days later.

Make a list of your favorite recipes and winning combinations so you can repeat them in the weeks that follow. As you experiment with new ingredients and dishes, add your successes to your list. Use whatever system works best for you, whether it's entering recipes in an electronic database, flagging pages with color-coded sticky notes, or simply writing notes in the margins of your cookbooks. By using some—or all—of these basic planning principles, you can count on quick and easy meals that are successful and stress free.

2 • shopping smart

With a weekly menu plan on paper and an organized shopping list in hand, you can greatly reduce your time at the grocery store *and* ensure that you get the most payback for your effort.

Once you've completed a written meal plan, list the ingredients you'll need for your chosen recipes for the timeframe you're working with. (We're assuming that you'll shop once a week to get the bulk of what you need, but your schedule may dictate otherwise.) Then check for the basics that you need to replace. The easiest way to keep track is to post a list where you can easily jot down an item *right when you think of it*. Do whatever works best for you, whether it's keeping a magnetized eraser board on the fridge or a list on your smartphone. The more efficient you are in your list making, the less time you'll waste on emergency trips to the store for a missing ingredient.

Once you're in the market, shop the perimeter of the store first—this is usually where you'll find the fresh foods, such as produce, meats, and dairy. Then move to the center aisles to pick up what's left on your list. As you shop, take advantage of the time-savers the store offers. For example, get ready-to-go salad fixings at the salad bar, buy peeled shrimp, and have the butcher debone or precut meats to your specifications.

As a general rule, it's best to be flexible but reasonable as you shop. It's great when sales and specials fit your plans, but don't forget to consider, for example, how quickly you'll use perishables like fruit and vegetables. No matter how good a deal is, you may end up with lots of waste if you can't use what you buy before it spoils.

STOCK UP ON THE BASICS

Keeping staples on hand gives you the ability to throw together a great, simple meal in a hurry. In fact, you'll be able to prepare most of the recipes in this book with the ingredients waiting in your well-equipped refrigerator, freezer, and pantry; for many other dishes, you'll need only a few additional items from the store.

Create an electronic list of these suggested basics, adding any favorites that are missing and deleting items you know you won't use. (You don't need to keep an overwhelming array of foods. Just add gradually to your stockpile until you reach the combination of staples that works best for you.) Each week, keep a running list of the things you've used up or that you want to add. For super-fast shopping, rearrange your list in order of how things are displayed in your favorite store so you'll be able to stock up efficiently and fast.

FRESH STAPLES
- ☐ onions
- ☐ garlic
- ☐ gingerroot
- ☐ lemons
- ☐ limes
- ☐ green chiles

STAPLES FOR THE FRIDGE
- ☐ shredded Parmesan cheese
- ☐ fat-free or low-fat Cheddar and Monterey Jack cheese (lowest sodium available)
- ☐ low-fat mozzarella cheese
- ☐ eggs
- ☐ egg substitute
- ☐ light tub margarine or fat-free spray margarine
- ☐ light mayonnaise
- ☐ fat-free milk
- ☐ fat-free yogurt: plain and sugar-free flavored

STAPLES FOR THE FREEZER
- ☐ chicken breasts
- ☐ fish fillets (individually wrapped)
- ☐ assorted vegetables without added sauces
- ☐ brown rice
- ☐ lean steaks and chops
- ☐ lean ground meat
- ☐ assorted fruits and berries

STAPLES FOR THE PANTRY

RICES
- ☐ instant and/or regular brown rice
- ☐ instant and/or regular white rice

BEANS
- ☐ no-salt-added canned kidney beans
- ☐ no-salt-added canned white beans
- ☐ no-salt-added canned black beans
- ☐ no-salt-added canned chickpeas
- ☐ dried beans, peas, and lentils

PASTAS AND GRAINS
- ☐ assorted whole-grain and enriched pastas
- ☐ oatmeal
- ☐ whole-wheat couscous
- ☐ barley
- ☐ bulgur
- ☐ quinoa

TOMATO PRODUCTS
- ☐ no-salt-added tomato sauce
- ☐ no-salt-added diced, stewed, and whole tomatoes
- ☐ no-salt-added tomato paste
- ☐ spaghetti sauces (lowest sodium available)

DRY GOODS

- [ ] flour—all-purpose and whole-wheat
- [ ] sugar—granulated, brown, and confectioners'
- [ ] baking soda
- [ ] baking powder
- [ ] cornstarch
- [ ] cornmeal
- [ ] plain dry bread crumbs
- [ ] panko (Japanese bread crumbs)

CANNED AND BOTTLED PRODUCTS

- [ ] fat-free, low-sodium broths
- [ ] low-sodium soups
- [ ] salmon and very low sodium tuna in water
- [ ] no-salt-added canned vegetables
- [ ] fruits canned in water or their own juice
- [ ] 100% fruit juices
- [ ] fat-free condensed milk
- [ ] roasted red bell peppers
- [ ] olives
- [ ] green chiles
- [ ] garlic—minced, chopped, or whole
- [ ] ginger, minced

COOKING OILS

- [ ] cooking sprays
- [ ] canola or corn oil
- [ ] olive oil
- [ ] toasted sesame oil

MISCELLANEOUS

- [ ] all-fruit spreads

- [ ] peanut butter (lowest sodium available)
- [ ] honey
- [ ] maple syrup
- [ ] unsalted nuts, such as almonds, walnuts, and pecans

CONDIMENTS
(choose lowest sodium available)

- [ ] vinegars
- [ ] mustards
- [ ] no-salt-added ketchup
- [ ] hoisin sauce
- [ ] red hot-pepper sauce
- [ ] salsa
- [ ] soy sauce
- [ ] teriyaki sauce
- [ ] Worcestershire sauce
- [ ] barbecue sauce

SPICES AND SEASONINGS

- [ ] dried herbs including oregano, basil, thyme, rosemary, dillweed
- [ ] garlic powder
- [ ] onion powder
- [ ] chili powder
- [ ] crushed red pepper flakes
- [ ] black pepper
- [ ] cayenne
- [ ] salt-free seasoning blends, such as Italian and all-purpose
- [ ] ground spices such as cinnamon, ginger, nutmeg, cumin, paprika
- [ ] salt
- [ ] vanilla extract

GET THE MOST FROM YOUR FRIDGE AND FREEZER

As you're thinking about how to shop smarter, be sure to incorporate the refrigerator and freezer into your planning. To start, create zones in your refrigerator so you can store each type of go-to staple in the area that will keep it fresh longest. In most refrigerators, the bottom and the back are the coolest areas and the door and the top are the warmest. Store dairy products, such as milk, in the middle of the fridge; keep the most perishable foods (fish or ground meat, for example) in the coldest spots or a meat drawer. The temperatures in the designated compartments on the door are just right for soft margarine and condiments.

Since, ideally, you'll be making your main shopping trip once a week, you can maximize prep time by washing, peeling, and chopping all your fresh produce at one convenient time—right after shopping, for example. Store the prepped food in separate airtight containers in the crisper; during the week, all you'll have to do is grab what you need.

Your freezer enables you to keep fish, meat, poultry, and lots of other staples on hand for quick, spur-of-the-moment meals. In theory, freezing keeps food safe to eat indefinitely, but it can also affect the quality and texture of food over time. When freezing foods, remember to date your containers for best results. For safe defrosting, thaw foods in the refrigerator, in cold water, or in the microwave, not at room temperature on the counter. (See Appendix C, "Food Safety Tips," for more information on how to keep your foods fresh and safe to eat.)

LEARN LABEL LINGO

To know what's really in the foods you buy, make it a habit to always check package labels, ingredient lists, and nutrition facts panels when you shop. It's also smart to be savvy about front-of-package labeling and marketing techniques; some claims can be misleading. For example, a product labeled "low-fat" may be very high in sodium or sugar instead.

The U.S. Food and Drug Administration and the U.S. Department of Agriculture regulate the information found on nutrition facts panels to help you compare products and make informed choices. Several organizations use their own icon systems to help you make decisions; some grocery stores are also using on-shelf labeling programs. The American Heart Association's heart-check mark is one example of reliable health labeling (see page 16 for more information on this program). When you see an

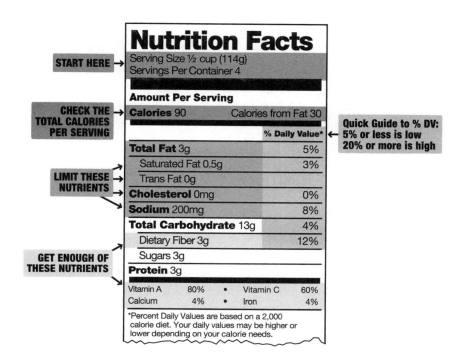

Nutrition Facts

START HERE → Serving Size ½ cup (114g)
Servings Per Container 4

Amount Per Serving

CHECK THE TOTAL CALORIES PER SERVING → **Calories** 90   Calories from Fat 30

Quick Guide to % DV: ← 5% or less is low
20% or more is high

% Daily Value*

Total Fat 3g	5%
Saturated Fat 0.5g	3%
Trans Fat 0g	
Cholesterol 0mg	0%
Sodium 200mg	8%
Total Carbohydrate 13g	4%
Dietary Fiber 3g	12%
Sugars 3g	
Protein 3g	

LIMIT THESE NUTRIENTS →

GET ENOUGH OF THESE NUTRIENTS →

Vitamin A	80%	Vitamin C	60%
Calcium	4%	Iron	4%

*Percent Daily Values are based on a 2,000 calorie diet. Your daily values may be higher or lower depending on your calorie needs.

icon or a health claim on food packaging, remember also to consider the information on the nutrition facts panel and the ingredient list before you select what to buy.

To read the nutrition facts panel, look at the serving size as it relates to the nutrient numbers. If, for example, the panel says the container holds two servings and you intend to eat the entire contents, you must double all the values and consider how they will add to your overall intake of calories, sodium, saturated fat, trans fat, and cholesterol. Keep in mind that for a 2,000-calorie diet, 40 calories per serving is considered low; 100 calories per serving, moderate; and 400 calories or more, high.

The % Daily Value column tells you the percentage of each nutrient in a single serving, based on the daily recommended amount. If you want to consume less of a nutrient, such as sodium, saturated fat, or cholesterol, choose foods with a lower % Daily Value (5% or less is considered low). If you want to consume more of a nutrient, such as fiber, look for foods with a higher % Daily Value (20% or more is considered high).

You can look to the American Heart Association Food Certification Program's heart-check mark to help you quickly find heart-healthy foods in the grocery store. When you see the heart-check mark on food packaging, you know that the product has been certified by the association to meet our criteria for foods that are higher sources of better fats but limited in saturated and trans fats, cholesterol, and sodium. To learn more, visit www.heartcheckmark.org. You'll also find a list of certified products and the free online "My Grocery List" builder, an easy-to-use tool to create and print a personalized heart-healthy shopping list.

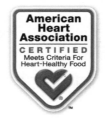

SHOP SMARTER FOR SNACKS

Snacks can help round out a healthy diet, but you need to be careful about what you select. There's an overwhelming array of snack choices, and some are better than others. Typically, the less processed a food, the less likely it is to be high in the dietary villains: sodium, unhealthy fats, and added sugars.

Manufacturers are creating many new packaged and frozen foods that cater to shoppers who are more health conscious. Just be sure to read nutrition facts panels carefully when you shop, since these products can vary widely in how well they adhere to heart-healthy guidelines. Making better choices also means replacing sugary beverages with flavored water, diet soda, or tea without added sugar. Instead of drinking fruit juices, eat whole fruit for the most health benefit. In fact, keeping fruit such as apples, grapes, and bananas on hand is a quick and easy way to satisfy a nagging sweet tooth without resorting to sugar-packed candies and desserts.

SHOP MENUS WHEN EATING OUT

Although you may have less control over food choices when you're eating in a restaurant or traveling, you still can select the healthiest options available. Read the restaurant menu for nutrition information, if possible. Many restaurants and chains provide this data online or make it available on-site. You can enjoy eating out *and* be good to your heart if you follow these suggestions:

- Watch portion size. Most restaurants serve much more food than you would normally eat at one meal. Put a reasonable portion of your entrée in a to-go box before you start to eat and take the rest home, or share with a friend.

- Choose the healthiest preparation method, such as grilled or broiled instead of fried.

- Ask for sauces and salad dressings on the side so you can control how much of them you eat.

- Make smart substitutions: For example, cut down on sodium and fat by swapping warm corn tortillas for fried tortilla chips.

- Research better choices at your favorite fast-food places. That way, when you do go, you'll know what to order. Buy just the foods you want rather than combo meals—remember, they aren't a good deal if you end up with lots of extra sodium, saturated fat, trans fat, cholesterol, and sugar!

3 • kitchen know-how

The following suggestions will help you get meals on the table faster and with little fuss. Spending a few minutes to get your kitchen organized and using savvy techniques for quicker cooking will save you valuable time in the long run.

GET ORGANIZED

The setup of your kitchen work areas can be the make-or-break element in your meal prep efficiency. Searching through cluttered cabinets and drawers saps time and energy and lessens the pleasure of cooking at home. It's well worth taking a little time up front to think through what works—and what doesn't. Every kitchen is unique, so be creative to find the best solutions for yours.

ORGANIZE YOUR SPACE
Take these steps to create customized efficiency in your kitchen:

- *Get rid of clutter.* Look through cabinets and drawers and assess what's on your countertops and in your pantry. Throw away or donate items that you haven't used at least once in the past year. If you just can't part with those items, move them to the garage or basement to save space for the things you use most often.

- *Reconsider your storage options.* Can you find a better way to organize and store things? For example, use mesh dividers to tame unruly cutlery and utensils in drawers. Hang pots and lids on walls or inside cupboard doors instead of stacking them. Store knives on a magnetic rack on the wall where you can reach them without effort. A magnetic rack also works well for often-used spices in metal containers. Put turntables or risers in cupboards so you can easily see what's there.

- *Designate areas for different tasks.* Choose a place for each job you do often: one for reading recipes, one for prep work, one for setting out ingredients, and so on. This will help you establish a routine that will make working in the kitchen go faster and smoother. If you adore baking, give the standing mixer a spot on the counter and put the bread machine where it's handy. On the other hand, if you need your blender only once a year, put it away and leave the more accessible space for the things you use more often.

- *Keep handy what you use every day.* You should be able to find knives, measuring spoons, whisks, and other basic utensils without rooting through a crowded drawer.

- *Group cooking equipment according to how it is used.* Store baking pans and baking sheets with muffin pans, put the roasting rack in the roasting pan, and keep the grilling tools and skewers together.

- *Organize your pantry, freezer, and fridge.* Using the same principle as for equipment, keep related foods together so you'll be able to quickly find the ingredient you need: Group canned vegetables together, soups together, and pastas and grains together, for example. If you have the space, alphabetize your spices.

- *Make it easy to get rid of food prep leftovers.* The peelings and other waste that are part of preparing food can accumulate quickly and clutter your workspace, but you don't want to have to walk across the kitchen every time you need to discard a potato peel. If you use a garbage disposal, make room to work by the sink; if you compost, keep a small bag or bowl on the counter to throw organics into and then transfer them to your compost when you are done.

- *Plan ahead for easy cleanup.* Set a thin plastic cutting board or a plate on your work surface. Put messy spoons and spatulas on it as you cook, and then just wash the board and utensils when you're ready. Line baking sheets with aluminum foil and fill dirty pots and pans with hot, soapy water right after you use them. You can also fill the sink or a large bowl with water and drop in dirty utensils (not knives or other sharp items). They'll be much easier to clean, especially if you need them again as you cook.

- *Control accumulation of storage items.* Use organizers to make it easy to store leftovers for another busy day. Stack plastic food containers with matching lids; throw away mismatched pieces. Mount dispensers on the wall or inside cabinet doors for plastic wrap, wax paper, and aluminum foil. Store plastic grocery bags in inexpensive hanging dispensers, or stuff the bags into empty paper towel tubes. To go green and cut down on the accumulation of all those bags, keep reusable cloth grocery bags in your car and use them instead.

ORGANIZE YOUR TOOLS

There's a right tool for every job, and every cook needs certain basic tools to cook efficiently. The following items are essential to a well-equipped kitchen:

- ☐ Several well-sharpened, high-quality knives
- ☐ A medium and a large skillet, each with a tight-fitting lid
- ☐ A covered pan you can use both on the stovetop and in the oven
- ☐ A few nonstick pots and pans
- ☐ Dutch oven
- ☐ A variety of covered casserole dishes
- ☐ Two dishwasher-safe chopping boards
- ☐ Food processor or blender
- ☐ A nest of mixing bowls
- ☐ A whisk, at least one big spoon and a slotted spoon, tongs, spatulas, and scrapers
- ☐ Kitchen scissors
- ☐ At least one set each of measuring spoons and measuring cups
- ☐ Vegetable peeler
- ☐ Can opener
- ☐ Colander
- ☐ A set of baking pans (including 8- or 9-inch square, 11 × 8 × 2-inch or 13 × 9 × 2-inch, and loaf) and a set of baking sheets
- ☐ Pot holders, trivets, and cooling racks
- ☐ Kitchen timer
- ☐ Grater
- ☐ Storage containers with lids
- ☐ Instant-read thermometer

Keep your tools and countertop appliances (blender, food processor) in good working order so you don't waste time. For example, dull knives will slow you down and make chopping more difficult, so it's worth the effort to keep knives sharpened. You'll always be ready for quick and easy prep work.

ORGANIZE YOUR APPROACH

When cooking from a recipe, be sure to read it all the way through first! You don't want to be caught halfway into preparing a dish only to find that you don't have a crucial ingredient or kitchen tool. Most professional chefs put out everything needed for a recipe, measured and ready to go (called *mise en place*), before they even turn on the stove or oven. Once you get used to this approach to cooking, you'll appreciate how much time it can save. Also, review the sequence of steps for things that can be done at the same time. For example, you can start boiling the pasta water while waiting for the onions to cook down for the sauce.

Most of all, try to stay flexible. It's great to cook fresh from scratch, but when time is short you may need to grab the dried minced onion instead. Stock up on "convenience" versions of the ingredients you use all the time, such as bottled minced garlic and ginger, bottled lemon and lime juice, and other basics that you can reach for when you just don't have time to mince, dice, or squeeze.

QUICK COOKING TECHNIQUES

When it comes to quick and easy recipes, both *how* you cook and *what* you cook determine the timeline. Some techniques are naturally fast and fuss free, and others allow you to walk away while food practically cooks itself. It's also important, of course, to choose a cooking method that's heart-healthy, as are all the techniques outlined below.

In general, the smaller the pieces of food, the faster they will cook through. Sautés and stir-fries are good examples of that principle. Grilling and broiling also work well with evenly sized, smaller portions, which is why many recipes for fish fillets, chicken breasts, and steaks call for these techniques. The slower methods, such as roasting and baking, require longer cooking times, but very often the preparation is so simple that you actually spend only minutes on each dish.

SPEEDY COOKING WITH SHORT PREP TIME

- *Broiling and Grilling.* The only real difference between these two fast-cooking methods is where the heat comes from: above the food in a broiler and below the food on a grill. The direct exposure to the heat browns the outside of the food while leaving the inside moist and tender. The food usually sits on a rack, which allows excess fat to drip away and air to circulate, helping food cook faster. Remember that if a broiling recipe specifies a distance from the heat, it means the number of inches from the heat element to the top of the food you are broiling, not to the top of the broiling rack. Try a variety of rubs, marinades, and glazes to add flavor; rubs in particular are super quick to use. To really make the most of the grill or broiler, cook vegetables and fruits along with meat, poultry, or seafood. The high heat caramelizes natural sugars and intensifies flavors.

- *Microwave Cooking.* Microwave ovens cook food by causing food molecules to vibrate, creating friction and therefore internal heat.

Because this method requires no added oils and very little, if any, liquid to keep food from drying out, it is a healthy way to prepare food. Probably the biggest benefit of cooking in a microwave oven is speed. As a rule of thumb, when microwaving, you can cut the cooking time to a third or even a quarter of the time in a conventional recipe. For example, you can microwave whole baking potatoes, pierced with a fork and wrapped in damp paper towels, in 10 minutes or less, which is about a quarter of the time it takes to bake them in the oven. If a food you are microwaving isn't done when you check it, *gradually* increase the cooking time until it is. Also, when converting most traditional recipes for the microwave, remember to reduce the amount of liquid by about one-third because less liquid evaporates during microwave cooking.

- *Sautéing and Stir-Frying.* Both sautéing and stir-frying involve quickly cooking food over direct heat, using a small amount of hot fat. Because the surface of meat, poultry, and seafood is seared over high heat at the outset with these techniques, the natural juices are sealed in, keeping the food moist. When sautéing, replace margarine with cooking spray to cut back on saturated fat, trans fat, and calories. Stir-frying moves fast. Because the heat is usually kept high throughout the cooking and little time is allowed between steps, prepare ingredients and sauces before you begin cooking.

- *Steaming.* Another quick and easy technique, steaming helps food retain flavor, color, and nutrients. Place the food in a basket over simmering liquid, making sure the liquid does not touch the bottom of the basket. For extra flavor, add onion, garlic, or herbs to the food or liquid. Most people are familiar with preparing vegetables this way, but remember that fish, chicken breasts, and any other foods that can be boiled or simmered are also excellent when steamed.

- *Poaching.* Poaching calls for immersing foods in almost-simmering liquid. This gentle technique is especially good for delicate foods, such as fish and fruit. Although you can use water as the cooking medium, most recipes for poaching use a liquid that adds flavor instead, such as wine or fat-free, low-sodium broth. After the food is cooked, remove it from the pan and reduce the remaining liquid (decrease the volume by boiling the liquid rapidly) to make a delicious sauce.

SLOWER COOKING WITH SHORT PREP TIME

- *Baking and Roasting.* Both baking and roasting use the dry heat of an oven to cook food. Depending on the size of the raw food, cooking time can range from 30 minutes to several hours. Except when making dishes that call for lots of ingredients (some lasagnas, for example), you don't need to spend much time preparing food to go into the oven. Many recipes just direct you to place seasoned food in a shallow baking pan, spray with cooking spray if needed, and cook until done. When baking coated fish fillets or chicken breasts, lightly mist with cooking spray. Although very simple once the food is in the oven, roasting typically requires a bit of preparation. Discard the visible fat and place meat or poultry on a rack in a roasting pan to prevent the food from sitting in its fat drippings. If needed, baste with fat-free liquids, such as wine, fruit juice, or fat-free, low-sodium broth. Plan on removing the food from the oven 15 to 20 minutes before serving. Letting the meat and poultry "rest" allows the juices to redistribute and makes carving easier. For whole birds, discard as much fat as you can before roasting, but to prevent dryness leave the skin on until the poultry is cooked. (Discard the skin before serving the poultry.) Save time and energy when the oven is on by roasting vegetables at the same time.

- *Braising and Stewing.* Although braised and stewed meats can take hours to reach fork-tender consistency, they don't usually take long to prep. The slow heat of both techniques breaks down less-tender cuts of meat and cooks fat out at the same time, so it's a good idea to cook ahead of time, refrigerate dishes overnight, and skim off and discard the hardened fat. Braises and stews are ideal to cook on a weekend, especially when you have a busy week ahead: The flavors of the foods blend and improve with time, and all you have to do on a hectic weeknight is reheat and serve.

- *Slow Cooking.* A slow cooker is designed to take the worry out of leaving food to cook while you are away from the kitchen. Just put food in the crock, cover it, and set the dial for high or low; some of the newer models can be set to turn off automatically or to switch from high to low or warm. You may also want to brown meats or poultry before adding them for color and deeper flavor. Don't fill the crock more than two-thirds full, layer ingredients as specified in the recipe, and don't open the cooker to stir, since removing the cover lets out heat and moisture. If a recipe makes more than you need right away, don't worry: Most slow-cooked meals are perfect for reheating later in the week.

TIPS FOR QUICKER COOKING

Several tricks of the trade can help you speed things up as you cook. Try these suggestions the next time you're cooking a meal.

- Cover Dutch ovens, stockpots, and saucepans to help liquids come to a boil faster; this is especially helpful when, for example, you need to boil water for pasta.

- Use wider skillets so that more liquid evaporates and food cooks more quickly.

- Choose thinner pastas when you're pressed for time; they cook more quickly than others. Angel hair and vermicelli give the speediest results; whole-grain pastas provide the most nutrients.

- Roast vegetables such as cauliflower, carrots, and onions while you roast or bake other foods. If you don't want to use the vegetables right away, freeze them for later use.

- Place your cutting board on a damp paper towel to keep the board from sliding.

- Grate cheese or lemon peel over a thin flexible cutting mat or wax paper. Then just bend the mat or paper and pour what you need into a measuring cup or spoon.

- Put small amounts of parsley, cilantro, and other herbs in a cup or small bowl and use kitchen scissors to snip them right there.

- Quickly peel fresh garlic with a garlic peeler (a rubber cylinder that rubs off the papery peel) or rubber jar opener. You can also smash garlic cloves with the flat of a knife; the skin will break apart.

- Measure dry ingredients before wet ones if the recipe allows so you can reuse measuring spoons and cups without having to wash them between steps.

- Spray utensils with cooking spray before measuring sticky ingredients such as honey or molasses. Cups and spoons will be much easier to clean.

- Make it much easier to thinly slice raw poultry or meat by first putting it in the freezer for 10 to 15 minutes.

- Microwave lemons and limes for about 10 seconds on 100 percent power (high) or roll them under your hand on a hard surface. Either technique makes them easier and faster to juice. Use what you need and freeze any extra juice by the tablespoonful in ice cube trays for quick access later on. You can also freeze extra lemon wedges or slices.

- Use a food processor or mandoline to make quick work of slicing and dicing in large quantities.

- Keep high-intensity, flavorful ingredients on hand. It takes no time to throw in a tablespoon of mint, unsalted pine nuts, or dried currants, any of which can make a simple dish outstanding.

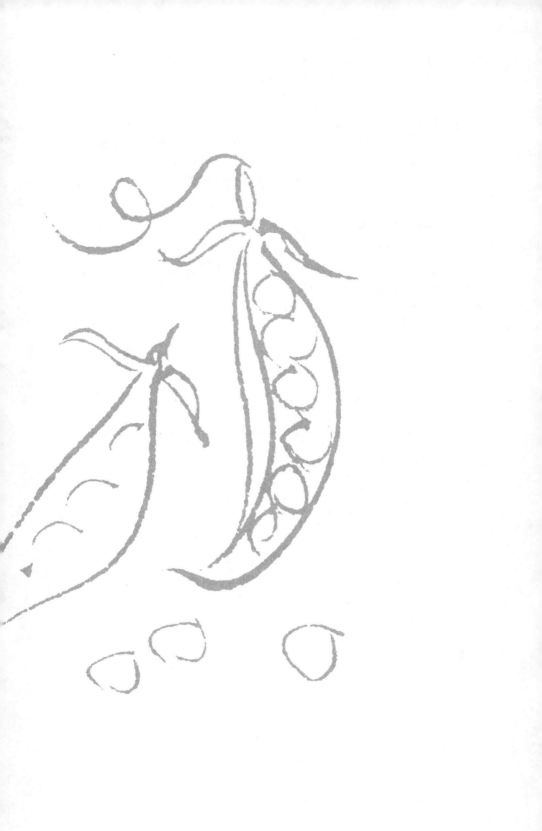

recipes

To help you plan meals and determine how a recipe fits into your overall eating plan, we have provided a nutrition analysis for each recipe in the book. The following guidelines give some details on how the analyses were calculated.

- Each analysis is for a single serving; garnishes or optional ingredients are not included unless noted.

- When figuring portions, remember that the serving sizes provided are approximate.

- When ingredient options are listed, the first one is analyzed. When a range of amounts is given, the average is analyzed.

- Values other than fats are rounded to the nearest whole number. Fat values are rounded to the nearest half gram. Because of the rounding, values for saturated, trans, polyunsaturated, and monounsaturated fats may not add up to the amount shown for total fat value.

- All the recipes are analyzed using unsalted or low-sodium ingredients whenever possible. In some cases, we call for unprocessed foods or no-salt-added and low-sodium products, then add table salt sparingly for flavor. If this book provides a recipe for a common ingredient, such as salsa, we use the data for our own version in the analysis and cross-reference the recipe. If only a regular commercial product is available, we use the one with the lowest sodium available.

- We specify canola, corn, and olive oils in these recipes, but you can also use other heart-healthy unsaturated oils, such as safflower, soybean, and sunflower.

- Meats are analyzed as lean, with all visible fat discarded. Values for ground beef are based on extra-lean meat that is 95 percent fat free.

- If meat, poultry, or seafood is marinated and the marinade is discarded, we calculate only the amount of marinade absorbed.

- If alcohol is used in a cooked dish, we estimate that most of the alcohol calories evaporate as the food cooks.

- Because product labeling in the marketplace can vary and change quickly, we use the generic terms "fat-free" and "low-fat" throughout to avoid confusion.

- We use the abbreviations "g" for gram and "mg" for milligram.

appetizers, snacks, and beverages

chickpea-pistachio dip

SERVES 7
¼ cup per serving

PREPARATION TIME
8 minutes

COOKING TIME
3 to 4 minutes

PER SERVING
Calories 106
Total Fat 2.5 g
  Saturated Fat 0.0 g
  Trans Fat 0.0 g
  Polyunsaturated Fat 0.5 g
  Monounsaturated Fat 1.0 g
Cholesterol 3 mg
Sodium 75 mg
Carbohydrates 16 g
  Fiber 3 g
  Sugars 2 g
Protein 5 g
Dietary Exchanges
  1 starch, ½ lean meat

Get this dip ready for your next snack attack! It's the perfect fit with fresh veggies or pieces of toasted whole-grain pita bread.

1   15.5-ounce can no-salt-added chickpeas, rinsed and drained
½   cup fat-free sour cream
2   medium green onions, chopped
3   tablespoons shelled pistachios, dry-roasted
2   tablespoons snipped fresh dillweed
1   tablespoon fresh lemon juice
1   tablespoon plain rice vinegar
1   teaspoon bottled minced garlic or 2 medium garlic cloves, minced
½   teaspoon olive oil (extra-virgin preferred)
½   teaspoon red hot-pepper sauce
⅛   teaspoon salt

In a food processor or blender, process all the ingredients for 20 seconds, or until almost smooth. Serve or refrigerate in an airtight container for up to two days.

edamame salsa

SERVES 8
¼ cup per serving

PREPARATION TIME
10 minutes

PER SERVING
Calories 37
Total Fat 2.0 g
  Saturated Fat 0.0 g
  Trans Fat 0.0 g
  Polyunsaturated Fat 0.0 g
  Monounsaturated Fat 1.0 g
Cholesterol 0 mg
Sodium 39 mg
Carbohydrates 3 g
  Fiber 1 g
  Sugars 2 g
Protein 2 g
Dietary Exchanges
  ½ fat

Serve this brightly colored, crunchy salsa as an appetizer with baked tortilla chips, such as Homemade Corn Tortilla Chips (page 40), or double the serving size and use it as a side salad.

¾ cup frozen shelled edamame, thawed and patted dry
 1 medium tomato, diced
½ medium cucumber, peeled and diced
½ to 1 medium fresh jalapeño, seeds and ribs discarded, finely chopped
¼ cup finely chopped red onion
 2 tablespoons snipped fresh mint
 2 teaspoons grated lemon zest
 2 tablespoons fresh lemon juice
 2 teaspoons olive oil (extra-virgin preferred)
⅛ teaspoon salt

In a medium bowl, gently stir together all the ingredients. Serve immediately for peak flavor.

COOK'S TIP ON HOT CHILE PEPPERS
Hot chile peppers, such as jalapeño, Anaheim, serrano, and poblano, contain oils that can burn your skin, lips, and eyes. Wear plastic gloves or wash your hands thoroughly with warm, soapy water immediately after handling hot peppers. Most of the spicy heat in a chile pepper, such as the jalapeño in this salsa, is found in the seeds and ribs (membranes). Leave them in for maximum heat; discard them if you prefer a milder flavor.

chunky salsa

SERVES 8
¼ cup per serving

PREPARATION TIME
7 minutes

Fresh bell pepper, green onions, and cilantro embellish canned tomatoes to make this salsa. Use it with Homemade Corn Tortilla Chips (page 40), over baked or grilled seafood or poultry, or even in place of salad dressing.

PER SERVING
Calories 16
Total Fat 0.0 g
  Saturated Fat 0.0 g
  Trans Fat 0.0 g
  Polyunsaturated Fat 0.0 g
  Monounsaturated Fat 0.0 g
Cholesterol 0 mg
Sodium 7 mg
Carbohydrates 3 g
  Fiber 1 g
  Sugars 2 g
Protein 1 g
Dietary Exchanges
  Free

- 1 **14.5-ounce can no-salt-added diced tomatoes, undrained**
- ½ **medium green or yellow bell pepper, chopped**
- 2 **medium green onions, sliced**
- 2 **tablespoons snipped fresh cilantro or parsley**
- 1 **tablespoon white wine vinegar**
- ½ **teaspoon ground cumin**
- ½ **teaspoon bottled minced garlic or 1 medium garlic clove, minced**
- ⅛ **teaspoon red hot-pepper sauce**

In a medium bowl, stir together all the ingredients. Serve or refrigerate in an airtight container for up to one week.

cranberry fruit dip

SERVES 4
¼ cup per serving

PREPARATION TIME
5 minutes

Pieces of fresh fruit, such as apple slices, orange sections, melon spears, and pineapple chunks, make tasty and attractive dippers for this refreshing dip.

PER SERVING
Calories 79
Total Fat 0.0 g
  Saturated Fat 0.0 g
  Trans Fat 0.0 g
  Polyunsaturated Fat 0.0 g
  Monounsaturated Fat 0.0 g
Cholesterol 1 mg
Sodium 29 mg
Carbohydrates 19 g
  Fiber 1 g
  Sugars 14 g
Protein 2 g
Dietary Exchanges
  1 other carbohydrate

- ½ **cup fat-free vanilla, lemon, or peach yogurt**
- ½ **cup whole-berry cranberry sauce**
- ¼ **teaspoon ground cinnamon**
- ⅛ **teaspoon ground ginger**

In a medium bowl, stir together all the ingredients. Serve or refrigerate in an airtight container for up to three days.

fruit kebabs

WITH HONEY-YOGURT DIP

SERVES 4
1 kebab and
2 tablespoons dip
per serving

PREPARATION TIME
10 to 12 minutes

PER SERVING
Calories 107
Total Fat 0.5 g
  Saturated Fat 0.0 g
  Trans Fat 0.0 g
  Polyunsaturated Fat 0.5 g
  Monounsaturated Fat 0.0 g
Cholesterol 1 mg
Sodium 26 mg
Carbohydrates 25 g
  Fiber 2 g
  Sugars 19 g
Protein 3 g
Dietary Exchanges
  1 fruit, ½ other
  carbohydrate

Let the kids skewer the fruit while you make the sweet and gingery dip for this great after-school snack.

DIP
- ½ cup fat-free plain yogurt
- 1 tablespoon honey
- 1 teaspoon poppy seeds
- ½ teaspoon vanilla extract
- ¼ teaspoon ground ginger

KEBABS
- 1 medium green kiwifruit, peeled and halved lengthwise, each half cut into 4 wedges
- 12 pineapple chunks, fresh or canned in their own juice, drained if canned
- 1 small banana, cut into 12 slices
- 12 red or green grapes, or a combination

In a small bowl, whisk together the dip ingredients. Set aside.

Using four 10-inch wooden skewers, thread in any order 2 kiwifruit wedges, 3 pineapple chunks, 3 banana slices, and 3 grapes on each. Serve the kebabs with the dip.

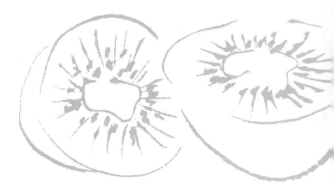

layered pesto spread

SERVES 4
3 tablespoons
per serving

PREPARATION TIME
8 to 10 minutes

CHILLING TIME
2 to 8 hours

PER SERVING
Calories 51
Total Fat 2.5 g
  Saturated Fat 0.5 g
  Trans Fat 0.0 g
  Polyunsaturated Fat 0.5 g
  Monounsaturated Fat 1.0 g
Cholesterol 4 mg
Sodium 149 mg
Carbohydrates 3 g
  Fiber 0 g
  Sugars 1 g
Protein 5 g
Dietary Exchanges
  1 lean meat

The layers of this impressive appetizer provide pleasing contrasts in both color and texture. Serve the spread with fat-free, low-sodium whole-grain crackers.

1 **cup fat-free cottage cheese**
2 **tablespoons Crunchy Basil-Parmesan Pesto (page 103) or commercial pesto**
  Paprika (optional)
  Several fresh basil leaves (optional)

Put the cottage cheese in a sieve. Drain well, using the back of a large spoon to press out as much liquid as possible. Transfer the cottage cheese to a food processor or blender. Process until smooth (there should be about ¾ cup).

Line a 1-cup custard cup or mold with plastic wrap. Spread ¼ cup cottage cheese over the bottom. Spread 1 tablespoon pesto over the cottage cheese. Repeat the layers, ending with the cottage cheese. Cover and refrigerate for 2 to 8 hours before serving.

At serving time, uncover the custard cup and invert the spread onto a serving plate. Remove the cup and carefully peel off the plastic wrap. Sprinkle the spread with the paprika. Garnish with the basil.

COOK'S TIP
If you don't have pesto left over from Baked Chicken with Crunchy Basil-Parmesan Pesto, you can make a batch in about 10 minutes. If you use commercial pesto, be aware that it is very likely to contain significantly more sodium and fat.

mushroom poppers

SERVES 8
4 pieces per serving

PREPARATION TIME
12 to 15 minutes

COOKING TIME
8 to 10 minutes

PER SERVING
Calories 44
Total Fat 1.0 g
  Saturated Fat 0.5 g
  Trans Fat 0.0 g
  Polyunsaturated Fat 0.0 g
  Monounsaturated Fat 0.0 g
Cholesterol 2 mg
Sodium 67 mg
Carbohydrates 6 g
  Fiber 1 g
  Sugars 1 g
Protein 4 g
Dietary Exchanges
  ½ starch

Parmesan, panko, and Italian herbs coat these moist mushroom morsels.

  2 **large egg whites**
  2 **teaspoons water**
  ⅔ **cup plain panko (Japanese bread crumbs)**
  ¼ **cup shredded or grated Parmesan cheese**
  1 **teaspoon dried Italian seasoning, crumbled**
  ½ **teaspoon dried basil, crumbled**
  ¼ **teaspoon pepper**
  1 **pound bite-size whole button mushrooms (about 32)**

Preheat the oven to 400°F.

In a small shallow dish, whisk together the egg whites and water.

In a large shallow dish, stir together the remaining ingredients except the mushrooms.

Put the dishes and a large baking sheet in a row, assembly-line fashion. Dip several mushrooms in the egg white mixture, turning to coat and letting any excess drip off. Dip in the panko mixture, turning to coat and gently shaking off any excess. Transfer to the baking sheet. Repeat with the remaining mushrooms, arranging in a single layer on the baking sheet.

Bake for 8 to 10 minutes, or until the coating is lightly browned.

COOK'S TIP ON CLEANING MUSHROOMS
To clean fresh mushrooms, wipe them with a clean, damp cloth or a mushroom brush. Gently pat them dry with paper towels. Because mushrooms absorb water like sponges, never soak them; you'll ruin their texture and taste.

mushroom quesadillas

SERVES 6
2 wedges per serving

PREPARATION TIME
6 to 8 minutes

COOKING TIME
10 to 12 minutes

OR

MICROWAVE TIME
6 to 9 minutes

PER SERVING

Calories 100
Total Fat 2.5 g
 Saturated Fat 1.0 g
 Trans Fat 0.0 g
 Polyunsaturated Fat 0.0 g
 Monounsaturated Fat 0.5 g
Cholesterol 5 mg
Sodium 212 mg
Carbohydrates 15 g
 Fiber 2 g
 Sugars 3 g
Protein 5 g
Dietary Exchanges
 1 starch, ½ fat

What makes these quesadillas so easy to prepare? You quickly cook a few ingredients, assemble the quesadillas, and bake or microwave them. If you wish, you can spoon a dollop of Chunky Salsa (page 32) on top. All that's left is to enjoy!

Cooking spray
8 ounces presliced button mushrooms (about 2½ cups)
½ medium onion, thinly sliced and separated into rings
1 teaspoon bottled minced garlic or 2 medium garlic cloves, minced
3 tablespoons snipped fresh cilantro
3 8-inch fat-free whole-wheat flour tortillas (lowest sodium available)
¼ cup plus 2 tablespoons shredded low-fat Monterey Jack cheese with jalapeño or low-fat Cheddar cheese

Preheat the oven to 350°F.

Lightly spray a large skillet with cooking spray. Cook the mushrooms, onion, and garlic over medium heat for 5 to 7 minutes, or until the onion is soft, stirring occasionally. Stir in the cilantro. Remove from the heat.

Spread the mushroom mixture on half of each tortilla. Sprinkle the Monterey Jack over the mushroom mixture. Fold the plain half of each tortilla over the filling. Transfer to a baking sheet.

Bake for 5 minutes, or until the filling is hot and the cheese has melted. Cut each quesadilla into 4 wedges. Serve warm.

MICROWAVE METHOD

Lightly spray a medium microwaveable glass dish with cooking spray. Microwave the mushrooms, onion, and garlic on 100 percent power (high) for 5 to 7 minutes, or until the onion is soft, stirring twice. Stir in the cilantro. Assemble the quesadillas as directed on page 36 and arrange on a microwaveable plate. Microwave on 100 percent power (high) for 1 to 2 minutes, or until the filling is hot and the cheese has melted. Cut each quesadilla into 4 wedges. Serve warm.

savory snack mix

SERVES 10
½ cup per serving

PREPARATION TIME
5 minutes

COOKING TIME
25 minutes

OR

MICROWAVE TIME
2 minutes

PER SERVING
Calories 73
Total Fat 3.0 g
   Saturated Fat 1.0 g
   Trans Fat 0.0 g
   Polyunsaturated Fat 0.5 g
   Monounsaturated Fat 1.5 g
Cholesterol 1 mg
Sodium 58 mg
Carbohydrates 9 g
   Fiber 0 g
   Sugars 0 g
Protein 2 g
Dietary Exchanges
   ½ starch, ½ fat

This five-ingredient nibble mix goes together in a snap, ready to bake or heat in a microwave whenever you crave a crunchy snack—fast!

6 4-inch rice or popcorn cakes, broken into bite-size pieces
2 cups bite-size low-sodium cheese-flavored or plain crackers (any shape)
2 tablespoons light tub margarine, melted
½ teaspoon chili powder
½ teaspoon garlic powder

Preheat the oven to 325°F.

Put the rice cakes and crackers in a large bowl.

In a small bowl, stir together the margarine, chili powder, and garlic powder. Pour over the rice-cake mixture, stirring to coat. Spread in a single layer on a baking sheet.

Bake for 25 minutes, stirring and turning over once or twice. Serve or let cool completely and store at room temperature in an airtight container for up to two weeks.

MICROWAVE METHOD

Combine the ingredients as directed above, transferring the mixture to a medium microwaveable bowl or casserole dish instead of a baking sheet. Microwave on 100 percent power (high) for 2 minutes, stirring once halfway through. Serve or store as directed.

sugar-and-spice snack mix

SERVES 14
½ cup per serving

PREPARATION TIME
5 minutes

COOKING TIME
25 minutes

OR

MICROWAVE TIME
3 minutes

COOLING TIME
10 minutes

PER SERVING
Calories 121
Total Fat 1.5 g
  Saturated Fat 0.0 g
  Trans Fat 0.0 g
  Polyunsaturated Fat 0.5 g
  Monounsaturated Fat 0.5 g
Cholesterol 0 mg
Sodium 79 mg
Carbohydrates 25 g
  Fiber 2 g
  Sugars 9 g
Protein 2 g
Dietary Exchanges
  1 starch, ½ fruit

Crisp and crunchy after it cools, this mix is perfect for an after-school snack or for packing in a lunch box.

3 cups lightly sweetened toasted oat squares cereal
3 cups miniature no-salt-added pretzels
2 tablespoons light tub margarine, melted
1 tablespoon firmly packed light brown sugar
½ teaspoon ground cinnamon
1 cup mixed dried fruit bits

Preheat the oven to 325°F.

Put the cereal and pretzels in a large bowl.

In a small bowl, stir together the margarine, brown sugar, and cinnamon. Pour over the cereal mixture, stirring to coat. Spread in a single layer on a large baking sheet.

Bake for 25 minutes, stirring and turning over once or twice.

Spread the mix on paper towels to cool for about 10 minutes. Transfer to an airtight container. Stir in the dried fruit. Serve or store at room temperature for up to two weeks.

MICROWAVE METHOD

Combine the ingredients as directed above, transferring the mixture to a medium microwaveable bowl or casserole dish instead of a baking sheet. Microwave on 100 percent power (high) for 3 minutes, stirring once every minute. Transfer to an airtight container. Stir in the dried fruit. Serve or store at room temperature for up to two weeks.

homemade corn tortilla chips

SERVES 8
5 chips per serving

PREPARATION TIME
5 minutes

COOKING TIME
8 to 10 minutes

PER SERVING
Calories 39
Total Fat 0.5 g
  Saturated Fat 0.0 g
  Trans Fat 0.0 g
  Polyunsaturated Fat 0.0 g
  Monounsaturated Fat 0.0 g
Cholesterol 0 mg
Sodium 101 mg
Carbohydrates 8 g
  Fiber 1 g
  Sugars 0 g
Protein 1 g
Dietary Exchanges
  ½ starch

By making your own chips, you can control how much sodium and fat they contain. Once the chips are baked, try adding a sprinkle of your favorite herb, spice, or salt-free seasoning blend for a change of flavor.

10 **6-inch corn tortillas**
    Cooking spray
¼ **teaspoon salt**

Preheat the oven to 400°F.

Place 3 or 4 tortillas in a stack. Cut the stack into 4 wedges. Repeat with the remaining tortillas, making a total of 40 wedges. Arrange in a single layer on 2 baking sheets. Lightly spray with cooking spray. Sprinkle with the salt.

Bake for 8 to 10 minutes, or until crisp. Serve, or if storing, transfer to cooling racks and let cool for 5 to 10 minutes. Store at room temperature in an airtight container for up to two weeks.

banana-kiwi smoothies

SERVES 2
1 cup per serving

PREPARATION TIME
5 minutes

PER SERVING
Calories 209
Total Fat 0.0 g
  Saturated Fat 0.0 g
  Trans Fat 0.0 g
  Polyunsaturated Fat 0.0 g
  Monounsaturated Fat 0.0 g
Cholesterol 4 mg
Sodium 111 mg
Carbohydrates 44 g
  Fiber 3 g
  Sugars 35 g
Protein 10 g
Dietary Exchanges
  1 fruit, 1 fat-free milk,
  1 other carbohydrate

Sweet and creamy, these smoothies provide both potassium and vitamin C.

1 **medium banana, quartered**
1 **medium kiwifruit, peeled and quartered**
1 **cup fat-free milk**
6 **ounces fat-free fruit-flavored yogurt**
2 **teaspoons sugar**

In a food processor or blender, process all the ingredients until smooth.

purple slurp

SERVES 4
1 cup per serving

PREPARATION TIME
5 minutes

PER SERVING
Calories 58
Total Fat 0.0 g
    Saturated Fat 0.0 g
    Trans Fat 0.0 g
    Polyunsaturated Fat 0.0 g
    Monounsaturated Fat 0.0 g
Cholesterol 0 mg
Sodium 34 mg
Carbohydrates 15 g
    Fiber 2 g
    Sugars 10 g
Protein 1 g
Dietary Exchanges
    1 fruit

CREAMY SLURP

Calories 93
Total Fat 0.0 g
    Saturated Fat 0.0 g
    Trans Fat 0.0 g
    Polyunsaturated Fat 0.0 g
    Monounsaturated Fat 0.0 g
Cholesterol 1 mg
Sodium 47 mg
Carbohydrates 22 g
    Fiber 2 g
    Sugars 17 g
Protein 2 g
Dietary Exchanges
    1 fruit, ½ other
    carbohydrate

Feel like a child again with every "slurp" you take of this fun and fruity concoction.

1½ cups fresh or frozen unsweetened mixed berries or whole hulled strawberries
 1 cup pomegranate juice (blueberry-pomegranate preferred)
 1 cup ice cubes
1½ cups diet ginger ale

In a blender, process the berries, juice, and ice cubes until smooth. Stir in the ginger ale. Serve immediately.

creamy slurp

In a blender, process ¾ cup fat-free vanilla frozen yogurt with the berries, juice, and ice cubes, as directed above. Reduce the amount of ginger ale to ¾ cup and stir it into the mixture. Serves 4; 1 cup per serving

COOK'S TIP
Don't add the ginger ale to the blender with the other ingredients. The carbonation will pop the top off the blender.

soups

skillet-roasted bell pepper, zucchini, and vermicelli soup

SERVES 4
1 cup per serving

PREPARATION TIME
8 to 10 minutes

COOKING TIME
13 to 15 minutes

PER SERVING
Calories 136
Total Fat 7.5 g
  Saturated Fat 1.0 g
  Trans Fat 0.0 g
  Polyunsaturated Fat 1.0 g
  Monounsaturated Fat 5.0 g
Cholesterol 0 mg
Sodium 124 mg
Carbohydrates 14 g
  Fiber 3 g
  Sugars 3 g
Protein 4 g
Dietary Exchanges
  ½ starch, 1 vegetable,
  1½ fat

There's no need to turn on the oven—and heat up your kitchen—to give vegetables that deep-roasted taste. Pull out your skillet instead, and let it do the work for you!

3   cups fat-free, low-sodium chicken broth
⅛ teaspoon crushed red pepper flakes
2   ounces uncooked whole-grain vermicelli or whole-grain thin spaghetti, broken into 2-inch pieces
1   teaspoon olive oil and 1 tablespoon plus 2 teaspoons olive oil (extra-virgin preferred), divided use
1   medium red bell pepper, chopped
1   medium zucchini, chopped
½ cup water
2   tablespoons chopped fresh basil or 2 teaspoons dried, crumbled
⅛ teaspoon salt

In a large saucepan, bring the broth and red pepper flakes to a boil over high heat. Stir in the pasta. Return to a boil. Reduce the heat and simmer, covered, for 10 minutes, or until the pasta is just tender.

Meanwhile, in a large nonstick skillet, heat 1 teaspoon oil over medium-high heat, swirling to coat the bottom. Cook the bell pepper and zucchini for 6 minutes, or until beginning to brown on the edges, stirring frequently. Remove from the heat.

Stir in the water, scraping the bottom and side of the skillet to dislodge any browned bits. Cover to keep the small amount of remaining liquid from evaporating. Set aside.

When the pasta is done, stir in the bell pepper mixture, basil, salt, and remaining 1 tablespoon plus 2 teaspoons oil.

puréed broccoli soup
WITH LEMON-INFUSED OIL

SERVES 4
1 scant cup per serving

PREPARATION TIME
8 minutes

COOKING TIME
6 to 7 minutes

PER SERVING
Calories 83
Total Fat 5.0 g
  Saturated Fat 0.5 g
  Trans Fat 0.0 g
  Polyunsaturated Fat 0.5 g
  Monounsaturated Fat 3.5 g
Cholesterol 0 mg
Sodium 151 mg
Carbohydrates 7 g
  Fiber 3 g
  Sugars 2 g
Protein 4 g
Dietary Exchanges
  1 vegetable, 1 fat

The secret is out! If you want a fresh new way to season soup, drizzle lemony olive oil on top. You'll get the tang in every spoonful.

TOPPING
- 1 tablespoon plus 1 teaspoon olive oil (extra-virgin preferred)
- 2 teaspoons grated lemon zest
- 1 tablespoon fresh lemon juice
- ⅛ teaspoon salt

- Cooking spray
- ¼ cup plus 2 tablespoons very finely chopped green onions and 2 tablespoons very finely chopped green onions, divided use
- 3 cups fat-free, low-sodium chicken broth
- 12 ounces fresh or frozen broccoli florets, thawed
- ⅛ teaspoon cayenne

In a small bowl, stir together the topping ingredients. Set aside.

Lightly spray a large saucepan with cooking spray. Cook ¼ cup plus 2 tablespoons green onions over medium-high heat for 1 minute, stirring once or twice.

Pour the broth into the pan. Increase the heat to high and bring the mixture to a boil. Stir in the broccoli and cayenne. Return to a boil. Reduce the heat and simmer, covered, for 2 to 3 minutes, or until the broccoli is just tender.

In a food processor or blender, process the soup in batches until smooth. Transfer to bowls.

Stir the topping mixture. Drizzle over each serving, but don't stir it into the soup. Sprinkle with the remaining 2 tablespoons green onions.

double-tomato soup

SERVES 6
heaping ¾ cup
per serving

PREPARATION TIME
10 minutes

COOKING TIME
22 minutes

PER SERVING
Calories 71
Total Fat 2.0 g
  Saturated Fat 0.5 g
  Trans Fat 0.0 g
  Polyunsaturated Fat 0.0 g
  Monounsaturated Fat 1.5 g
Cholesterol 1 mg
Sodium 56 mg
Carbohydrates 10 g
  Fiber 2 g
  Sugars 6 g
Protein 2 g
Dietary Exchanges
  2 vegetable, ½ fat

This soup gets a double punch of flavor from sun-dried and canned tomatoes.

2   teaspoons olive oil
1   small carrot, chopped
1   small rib of celery, chopped
¼   cup chopped onion
½   teaspoon bottled minced garlic or 1 medium garlic clove, minced
2   14.5-ounce cans no-salt-added diced tomatoes, undrained
2   cups water
8   dry-packed sun-dried tomato halves, chopped
⅛   teaspoon dried oregano, crumbled
⅛   teaspoon dried basil, crumbled
    Pinch of pepper
2   tablespoons shredded or grated Parmesan cheese

In a large saucepan, heat the oil over medium-high heat, swirling to coat the bottom. Cook the carrot, celery, onion, and garlic for 3 minutes, stirring frequently.

Stir in the remaining ingredients except the Parmesan. Increase the heat to high and bring to a boil. Reduce the heat and simmer, covered, for 15 minutes, or until the vegetables are tender. Serve the soup sprinkled with the Parmesan.

COOK'S TIP ON SUN-DRIED TOMATOES
Dry-packed sun-dried tomatoes have a fresher tomato flavor and fewer calories than those packed in oil. If you can't find the dry-packed kind, you can substitute oil-packed, but be sure to blot them well with paper towels before chopping.

spinach and brown rice soup
WITH GINGER

SERVES 6
¾ cup per serving

PREPARATION TIME
13 minutes

COOKING TIME
4 minutes

PER SERVING
Calories 59
Total Fat 1.0 g
  Saturated Fat 0.0 g
  Trans Fat 0.0 g
  Polyunsaturated Fat 0.0 g
  Monounsaturated Fat 0.0 g
Cholesterol 10 mg
Sodium 114 mg
Carbohydrates 7 g
  Fiber 1 g
  Sugars 0 g
Protein 6 g
Dietary Exchanges
  ½ starch, ½ very lean meat

Serve this delicate, aromatic soup as a starter course or side dish, or pair it with spring greens and fruit salad for a light lunch.

  3   cups fat-free, low-sodium chicken broth
  5   ounces frozen cooked brown rice (about 1 cup)
  2   teaspoons bottled minced garlic or 4 medium garlic cloves, minced
  ¼   teaspoon crushed red pepper flakes
  ¾   ounce spinach, coarsely chopped (about ¾ cup)
  ½   cup diced cooked chicken breast, cooked without salt
  ½   cup finely chopped yellow bell pepper
  3   tablespoons chopped fresh basil (optional)
  1   tablespoon minced peeled gingerroot
  1   teaspoon soy sauce (lowest sodium available)
  ⅛   teaspoon salt
  ½   cup snipped fresh cilantro or finely chopped green onions (cilantro preferred)

In a large saucepan, bring the broth, rice, garlic, and red pepper flakes to a boil over high heat. Remove from the heat.

Stir in the remaining ingredients except the cilantro. Sprinkle with the cilantro.

COOK'S TIP ON SOY SAUCE
Different brands of soy sauce can vary widely in sodium content. When you shop for this classic ingredient, be sure to compare the nutrition facts panels of the available brands and pick the one with the least sodium.

mushroom-asparagus chowder

SERVES 6
heaping ¾ cup
per serving

PREPARATION TIME
7 minutes

COOKING TIME
15 minutes

PER SERVING
Calories 98
Total Fat 0.5 g
  Saturated Fat 0.0 g
  Trans Fat 0.0 g
  Polyunsaturated Fat 0.0 g
  Monounsaturated Fat 0.0 g
Cholesterol 3 mg
Sodium 204 mg
Carbohydrates 16 g
  Fiber 2 g
  Sugars 9 g
Protein 9 g
Dietary Exchanges
  ½ fat-free milk, 1 vegetable

Fat-free evaporated milk combined with a small amount of flour replaces the heavy cream that often provides chowders with their thickness. Who needs all those extra calories and grams of saturated fat and cholesterol?

3 cups fat-free, low-sodium chicken broth
¼ teaspoon salt
¼ teaspoon ground nutmeg
⅛ teaspoon pepper
1 pound asparagus, trimmed and cut on the diagonal into 1-inch pieces
8 ounces presliced button mushrooms (about 2½ cups)
12 ounces fat-free evaporated milk
¼ cup all-purpose flour

In a large saucepan, bring the broth, salt, nutmeg, and pepper to a boil over high heat.

Stir in the asparagus and mushrooms. Return to a boil. Reduce the heat and simmer, covered, for 5 minutes, or until the asparagus is just tender.

Meanwhile, in a small bowl, whisk together the milk and flour. When the asparagus is ready, pour the milk mixture into the soup.

Cook over medium heat for 6 minutes, or until thickened and bubbly, stirring frequently.

peppery pumpkin soup

SERVES 6
2/3 cup per serving

PREPARATION TIME
5 minutes

COOKING TIME
15 minutes

PER SERVING
Calories 87
Total Fat 0.5 g
  Saturated Fat 0.0 g
  Trans Fat 0.0 g
  Polyunsaturated Fat 0.0 g
  Monounsaturated Fat 0.0 g
Cholesterol 4 mg
Sodium 145 mg
Carbohydrates 15 g
  Fiber 3 g
  Sugars 10 g
Protein 7 g
Dietary Exchanges
  ½ starch, ½ fat-free milk

You don't need to wait until pumpkin harvest to try this first-course soup. Because it's made with canned pumpkin, you can enjoy it all year long.

- 1 **15-ounce can solid-pack pumpkin (not pie filling)**
- 1¼ **cups fat-free, low-sodium chicken broth**
- ¼ **teaspoon onion powder**
- ⅛ to ¼ **teaspoon pepper**
- ⅛ **teaspoon salt**
- ⅛ **teaspoon ground nutmeg**
- 1 **12-ounce can fat-free evaporated milk**
- ¼ **cup fat-free sour cream**
- 1 **tablespoon unsalted shelled pumpkin seeds (optional)**

In a medium saucepan, stir together the pumpkin, broth, onion powder, pepper, salt, and nutmeg. Cook over medium-high heat for 10 minutes, or until bubbly, stirring occasionally.

Stir in the milk. Cook for 5 minutes, or until heated through; don't let the soup come to a boil. Serve with dollops of sour cream and a sprinkling of pumpkin seeds.

chilled strawberry-cantaloupe soup

SERVES 4
¾ cup per serving

PREPARATION TIME
10 minutes

PER SERVING
Calories 102
Total Fat 0.5 g
 Saturated Fat 0.0 g
 Trans Fat 0.0 g
 Polyunsaturated Fat 0.0 g
 Monounsaturated Fat 0.0 g
Cholesterol 1 mg
Sodium 34 mg
Carbohydrates 23 g
 Fiber 2 g
 Sugars 18 g
Protein 3 g
Dietary Exchanges
 1½ fruit

Serve this soup as a delicious addition to breakfast or brunch, or pair it with Tuna Salad Bundles with Lemon and Dill (page 64) for a light summery lunch.

 ½ **medium cantaloupe, cut into chunks (about 2 cups), chilled**
 1 **cup hulled strawberries or raspberries, chilled**
 1 **small banana, cut into chunks**
 ½ **cup unsweetened pineapple juice, chilled**
 ½ **cup fat-free vanilla yogurt, chilled**

In a food processor or blender, process all the ingredients except the yogurt until smooth.

Add the yogurt. Process until combined. Serve or refrigerate in an airtight container for up to 24 hours.

curried shrimp bisque

SERVES 6
scant 1½ cups per serving

PREPARATION TIME
15 to 20 minutes

COOKING TIME
23 to 28 minutes

PER SERVING
Calories 196
Total Fat 1.0 g
  Saturated Fat 0.5 g
  Trans Fat 0.0 g
  Polyunsaturated Fat 0.5 g
  Monounsaturated Fat 0.0 g
Cholesterol 112 mg
Sodium 304 mg
Carbohydrates 31 g
  Fiber 3 g
  Sugars 11 g
Protein 18 g
Dietary Exchanges
  1½ starch, ½ fruit,
  2 very lean meat

Shrimp lovers will rejoice when they taste this bisque, which is deep golden in color, rich with curry flavor, and loaded with shrimp.

Cooking spray
2   medium apples, peeled and chopped
1   cup chopped onion
½   cup preshredded carrot
1   medium rib of celery, sliced
2   cups fat-free, low-sodium chicken broth
2   medium baking potatoes, peeled and diced
2   tablespoons curry powder
¼   teaspoon ground cardamom
¼   teaspoon ground allspice
¼   teaspoon salt
1   cup fat-free half-and-half
¼   cup no-salt-added tomato sauce
1   pound frozen peeled raw medium shrimp, rinsed
    Snipped fresh cilantro (optional)

Lightly spray a large saucepan with cooking spray. Cook the apples, onion, carrot, and celery over medium-high heat for 5 minutes, or until the apples are tender, stirring frequently.

Stir in the broth, potatoes, curry powder, cardamom, allspice, and salt. Bring to a boil. Reduce the heat and simmer, covered, for 10 minutes, or until the potatoes are tender.

In a food processor or blender, process the soup plus the half-and-half and tomato sauce in batches until smooth. Return the soup to the pan.

Bring the soup to a boil over high heat. Stir in the shrimp. Reduce the heat and simmer for 3 to 5 minutes, or until the shrimp are pink. Serve garnished with the cilantro.

COOK'S TIP
You can make this soup in advance and refrigerate it right after pureeing. Just before serving, bring the soup to a boil, add the shrimp, and finish cooking as directed.

thirty-minute minestrone

SERVES 8
1¼ cups per serving

PREPARATION TIME
15 minutes

COOKING TIME
15 minutes

PER SERVING
Calories 128
Total Fat 1.0 g
  Saturated Fat 0.5 g
  Trans Fat 0.0 g
  Polyunsaturated Fat 0.0 g
  Monounsaturated Fat 0.5 g
Cholesterol 2 mg
Sodium 128 mg
Carbohydrates 23 g
  Fiber 5 g
  Sugars 7 g
Protein 6 g
Dietary Exchanges
  1 starch, 2 vegetable

Although the list of ingredients for this classic Italian soup is long, the preparation is easy.

4　cups water
2　cups baby carrots
1　15.5-ounce can reduced-sodium Great Northern beans, rinsed and drained
1　14.5-ounce can no-salt-added diced tomatoes, undrained
1　cup chopped onion
1　tablespoon plus 1 teaspoon very low sodium beef bouillon granules
1　teaspoon bottled minced garlic or 2 medium garlic cloves, minced
½　teaspoon dried basil, crumbled
½　teaspoon dried oregano, crumbled
½　teaspoon pepper
9　or 10 ounces frozen Italian green beans
1　small zucchini, halved lengthwise and sliced crosswise
½　cup dried whole-grain elbow macaroni or broken dried whole-grain spaghetti
¼　cup shredded or grated Parmesan cheese

In a large saucepan, stir together the water, carrots, Great Northern beans, tomatoes with liquid, onion, bouillon granules, garlic, basil, oregano, and pepper. Bring to a boil over high heat.

Stir in the green beans, zucchini, and pasta. Return to a boil. Reduce the heat and simmer, covered, for 10 minutes, or until the pasta is tender. Serve sprinkled with the Parmesan.

rosemary-lemon vegetable soup

SERVES 4
1½ cups per serving

PREPARATION TIME
12 to 15 minutes

COOKING TIME
24 minutes

PER SERVING
Calories 266
Total Fat 3.5 g
  Saturated Fat 0.5 g
  Trans Fat 0.0 g
  Polyunsaturated Fat 1.0 g
  Monounsaturated Fat 1.0 g
Cholesterol 0 mg
Sodium 269 mg
Carbohydrates 48 g
  Fiber 9 g
  Sugars 12 g
Protein 11 g
Dietary Exchanges
  2 starch, 3 vegetable

Amaranth, considered a supergrain, combines with red beans to contribute the protein in this dish. If you have cooked amaranth before, this soup will be a nutritious addition to your repertoire; if you haven't, it will be an easy introduction to a different whole grain.

1 teaspoon olive oil
1 medium onion, chopped
1 teaspoon bottled minced garlic or 2 medium garlic cloves, minced
2 14.5-ounce cans no-salt-added diced tomatoes, undrained
1 15.5-ounce can no-salt-added small red beans, rinsed and drained
2 cups low-sodium vegetable broth
1 large carrot, chopped
1 medium rib of celery, chopped
½ cup uncooked amaranth
2 tablespoons no-salt-added tomato paste
2 teaspoons finely snipped fresh rosemary
1 teaspoon grated lemon zest
2 teaspoons fresh lemon juice
¼ teaspoon pepper
¼ teaspoon salt

In a large saucepan, heat the oil over medium-high heat, swirling to coat the bottom. Cook the onion for 2 minutes, or until almost soft, stirring frequently.

Stir in the garlic. Cook for 1 minute, stirring frequently.

Stir in the tomatoes with liquid, beans, broth, carrot, celery, amaranth, and tomato paste. Bring to a boil, still over medium-high heat. Reduce the heat and simmer, covered, for 15 minutes, or until the amaranth is tender. Remove from the heat.

Stir in the remaining ingredients. Serve immediately so the amaranth doesn't continue to absorb liquid and make the soup too thick.

COOK'S TIP ON AMARANTH

Amaranth is a tiny grain with a mild flavor similar to that of quinoa. Amaranth cooks quickly, making it a great choice when you're trying to fit more whole grains into your busy schedule. A source of fiber and protein and the only grain that contains a good amount of calcium, amaranth is available in some supermarkets and in health food stores.

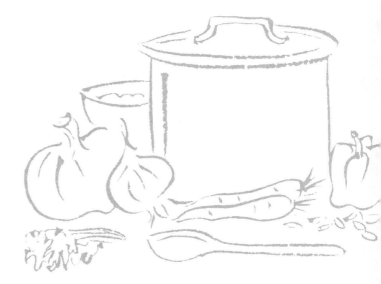

beef and vegetable soup
WITH CILANTRO AND LIME

SERVES 4
1¾ cups per serving

PREPARATION TIME
10 to 12 minutes

COOKING TIME
21 minutes

PER SERVING
Calories 178
Total Fat 3.5 g
  Saturated Fat 1.0 g
  Trans Fat 0.0 g
  Polyunsaturated Fat 0.5 g
  Monounsaturated Fat 1.5 g
Cholesterol 31 mg
Sodium 175 mg
Carbohydrates 20 g
  Fiber 3 g
  Sugars 6 g
Protein 17 g
Dietary Exchanges
  ½ starch, 2 vegetable,
  2 lean meat

The last-minute addition of snipped cilantro and a splash of lime juice really brighten the flavor of this vegetable-packed soup. Serve it with Easy Mexican Cornbread (page 231) for a satisfying meal.

8 ounces extra-lean ground beef
1 small carrot, chopped
1 small onion, chopped
2 teaspoons ground cumin
½ teaspoon dried oregano, crumbled
½ teaspoon bottled minced garlic or 1 medium garlic clove, minced
⅛ teaspoon cayenne
3½ cups fat-free, no-salt-added beef broth
1 14.5-ounce can no-salt-added diced tomatoes, undrained
½ cup uncooked instant brown rice
1 small yellow summer squash, chopped
¼ cup snipped fresh cilantro
2 tablespoons fresh lime juice

In a large saucepan, cook the beef, carrot, onion, cumin, oregano, garlic, and cayenne over medium-high heat for 8 minutes, or until the beef is browned on the outside and no longer pink in the center, stirring occasionally to turn and break up the beef.

Stir in the broth, tomatoes with liquid, and rice. Increase the heat to high and bring to a boil. Reduce the heat and simmer, covered, for 5 minutes.

Stir in the squash and simmer, covered, for 5 minutes, or until the squash is tender-crisp. Stir in the cilantro and lime juice.

salads

strawberry-spinach salad
WITH CHAMPAGNE DRESSING

SERVES 4
1¼ cups per serving

PREPARATION TIME
15 minutes

COOKING TIME
3 to 4 minutes

PER SERVING
Calories 94
Total Fat 4.5 g
  Saturated Fat 0.5 g
  Trans Fat 0.0 g
  Polyunsaturated Fat 1.0 g
  Monounsaturated Fat 2.5 g
Cholesterol 0 mg
Sodium 29 mg
Carbohydrates 11 g
  Fiber 3 g
  Sugars 6 g
Protein 3 g
Dietary Exchanges
  1 fruit, 1 fat

This vibrantly colored salad complements almost any entrée. Just a few of the many possibilities are Dilled Albacore Cakes (page 94), Lemon-Pepper Chicken over Pasta (page 112), Sliced Sirloin with Leek Sauce (page 146), and Greek Omelet (page 195).

DRESSING
- **3 tablespoons brut champagne, champagne vinegar, or white wine vinegar**
- **1 tablespoon all-fruit strawberry spread**
- **1 teaspoon canola or corn oil**

SALAD
- **5 ounces spinach, torn into bite-size pieces (about 5 cups)**
- **2 cups halved hulled strawberries**
- **¼ cup sliced almonds, dry-roasted**

In a small bowl, whisk together the dressing ingredients.

In a large bowl, gently toss together the spinach and strawberries. Pour the dressing over the salad, gently tossing to coat. Sprinkle with the almonds.

COOK'S TIP ON DRY-ROASTING NUTS
Put the nuts in a single layer in a small skillet. Dry-roast over medium heat for 3 to 4 minutes, or until just fragrant, stirring frequently.

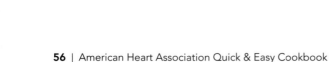

mustard-marinated vegetable salad

Vegetables marinate in a tangy citrus dressing flavored with tarragon and marjoram for a perfect side salad.

SALAD
14 to 16 ounces frozen mixed vegetables, such as cauliflower florets, baby brussels sprouts, broccoli florets, and carrots
1 small yellow summer squash, sliced (optional)

DRESSING
3 tablespoons fresh orange juice
2 tablespoons cider vinegar
1½ tablespoons olive oil (extra-virgin preferred)
1 tablespoon Dijon mustard (lowest sodium available)
½ teaspoon bottled minced garlic or 1 medium garlic clove, minced
¼ teaspoon dried tarragon, crumbled
¼ teaspoon dried marjoram, crumbled
¼ teaspoon salt
⅛ teaspoon pepper

In a medium glass dish, such as an 8-inch square, stir together the salad ingredients, breaking them apart if necessary.

In a small bowl, whisk together the dressing ingredients. Pour over the vegetables, tossing to coat. Let stand, covered, at room temperature for 3 hours to 3 hours 30 minutes, or until the frozen vegetables are thawed, stirring occasionally. If you prefer to serve the salad chilled, refrigerate for about 30 minutes, continuing to stir occasionally.

COOK'S TIP
If you want to make the salad a day in advance, refrigerate the covered vegetables and let thaw overnight, stirring occasionally.

no-chop cajun coleslaw

SERVES 6
½ cup per serving

PREPARATION TIME
5 minutes

CHILLING TIME
2 to 24 hours

PER SERVING
Calories 63
Total Fat 4.5 g
  Saturated Fat 0.5 g
  Trans Fat 0.0 g
  Polyunsaturated Fat 3.5 g
  Monounsaturated Fat 1.0 g
Cholesterol 7 mg
Sodium 193 mg
Carbohydrates 5 g
  Fiber 1 g
  Sugars 2 g
Protein 1 g
Dietary Exchanges
  1 vegetable, 1 fat

By using bagged cabbage and carrot slaw, you can put this spicy salad together in just 5 minutes. All that's left is to chill it and enjoy!

5 cups packaged shredded cabbage and carrot slaw
½ cup light mayonnaise
1 tablespoon white wine vinegar or cider vinegar
2 teaspoons bottled white horseradish, drained
¼ teaspoon onion powder
⅛ teaspoon cayenne

Put the slaw in a large bowl.

In a small bowl, whisk together the remaining ingredients. Pour over the slaw, tossing to coat. Cover and refrigerate for 2 to 24 hours. Stir just before serving.

grilled pineapple
WITH ZESTY BLUEBERRY TOPPING

SERVES 4
1 pineapple slice and
¼ cup berry mixture
per serving

PREPARATION TIME
8 minutes

COOKING TIME
6 minutes

COOLING TIME
8 to 10 minutes

PER SERVING
Calories 62
Total Fat 0.0 g
 Saturated Fat 0.0 g
 Trans Fat 0.0 g
 Polyunsaturated Fat 0.0 g
 Monounsaturated Fat 0.0 g
Cholesterol 0 mg
Sodium 1 mg
Carbohydrates 16 g
 Fiber 2 g
 Sugars 12 g
Protein 1 g
Dietary Exchanges
 1 fruit

Blending the sweetness of grilled pineapple and the zing of blueberries with raspberry vinegar and orange zest, this so-easy salad is the perfect accent for grilled entrées.

   Cooking spray
4 ½-inch-thick slices of fresh pineapple
2 tablespoons raspberry vinegar
2 teaspoons sugar
1 teaspoon grated orange zest
1 cup fresh or frozen blueberries, thawed and
   patted dry if frozen
2 tablespoons finely chopped red onion

Lightly spray the grill rack with cooking spray. Preheat the grill on medium high.

Lightly spray both sides of the pineapple with cooking spray.

Grill the pineapple for 3 minutes on each side, or until tender and beginning to richly brown. Transfer to a large plate. Refrigerate for 8 to 10 minutes to cool quickly, turning once halfway through.

Meanwhile, in a small bowl, stir together the vinegar, sugar, and orange zest until the sugar is dissolved. Gently stir in the blueberries and onion. Spoon over the chilled pineapple.

pasta and sugar snap pea salad

SERVES 4
½ cup per serving

PREPARATION TIME
10 to 12 minutes

COOKING TIME
20 minutes

PER SERVING
Calories 77
Total Fat 1.5 g
  Saturated Fat 0.0 g
  Trans Fat 0.0 g
  Polyunsaturated Fat 0.5 g
  Monounsaturated Fat 1.0 g
Cholesterol 0 mg
Sodium 67 mg
Carbohydrates 13 g
  Fiber 2 g
  Sugars 2 g
Protein 3 g
Dietary Exchanges
  1 starch

Don't let the penne in this recipe fool you—this salad is definitely Asian-inspired. Use it to complement Marinated Hoisin Chicken (page 100) or Chinese-Style Chicken (page 104), or turn it into a main dish by adding unsalted cooked shrimp or chicken.

2 ounces dried whole-grain penne (scant ¾ cup)
3 ounces sugar snap peas, trimmed (about 1 cup)
2 teaspoons soy sauce (lowest sodium available)
2 teaspoons plain rice vinegar
1 teaspoon canola or corn oil
¼ teaspoon grated peeled gingerroot
¼ medium red bell pepper, cut into short, thin strips
¼ small red onion, thinly sliced
1 tablespoon snipped fresh cilantro

Prepare the pasta using the package directions, omitting the salt and adding the peas during the last 2 minutes of cooking time. Transfer to a colander. Run under cold water for 1 to 2 minutes, or until cool. Drain well. Set aside.

Meanwhile, in a small bowl, whisk together the soy sauce, vinegar, oil, and gingerroot. Set aside.

In a large bowl, stir together the bell pepper, onion, and cilantro. Set aside.

When the pasta mixture is cool, stir in the bell pepper mixture. Pour in the dressing, tossing to coat. Serve at room temperature for the best flavor.

COOK'S TIP
If you refrigerate this salad longer than 4 hours, the vinegar will make the peas look unappealing.

fresh herb potato salad

SERVES 6
½ cup per serving

PREPARATION TIME
15 minutes

CHILLING TIME
2 to 24 hours

PER SERVING

Calories 84
Total Fat 2.5 g
  Saturated Fat 0.0 g
  Trans Fat 0.0 g
  Polyunsaturated Fat 2.0 g
  Monounsaturated Fat 0.5 g
Cholesterol 3 mg
Sodium 133 mg
Carbohydrates 14 g
  Fiber 3 g
  Sugars 2 g
Protein 2 g
Dietary Exchanges
  1 starch, ½ fat

Although this salad uses canned potatoes for speedy preparation, it gets a lot of fresh flavor from carrot, celery, dillweed, and basil.

1　**15-ounce can no-salt-added whole potatoes, rinsed, drained, patted dry, and cut into bite-size pieces**

1　**medium carrot, sliced**

1　**medium rib of celery, sliced**

½　**cup frozen green peas (tiny preferred)**

1　**tablespoon chopped shallot or green onion**

¼　**cup light mayonnaise**

1½　**teaspoons snipped fresh dillweed or ¼ teaspoon dried, crumbled**

1½　**teaspoons snipped fresh basil or ¼ teaspoon dried, crumbled**

1　**teaspoon Dijon mustard (lowest sodium available)**

1　**teaspoon white wine vinegar**
　　Pinch of pepper

In a large bowl, stir together the potatoes, carrot, celery, peas, and shallot.

In a small bowl, whisk together the remaining ingredients. Pour over the potato mixture, stirring to coat. Cover and refrigerate for 2 to 24 hours. Stir just before serving.

mediterranean black bean salad

SERVES 6
½ cup per serving

PREPARATION TIME
15 minutes

CHILLING TIME
2 to 24 hours

PER SERVING
Calories 84
Total Fat 1.0 g
 Saturated Fat 0.0 g
 Trans Fat 0.0 g
 Polyunsaturated Fat 0.0 g
 Monounsaturated Fat 0.5 g
Cholesterol 0 mg
Sodium 5 mg
Carbohydrates 15 g
 Fiber 4 g
 Sugars 4 g
Protein 5 g
Dietary Exchanges
 1 starch

Balsamic vinegar gives a slightly sweet-tart flavor to this version of black bean salad.

1   **15.5-ounce can no-salt-added black beans, rinsed and drained**
1   **medium red, yellow, or orange bell pepper, chopped**
1   **medium green bell pepper, chopped**
2   **tablespoons chopped onion**
2   **tablespoons fat-free, low-sodium chicken broth**
1   **tablespoon balsamic vinegar or red wine vinegar**
1   **teaspoon olive oil (extra-virgin preferred)**
½   **teaspoon bottled minced garlic or 1 medium garlic clove, minced**
¼   **teaspoon dried thyme, crumbled**
¼   **teaspoon dried rosemary, crushed**
⅛   **teaspoon pepper**
¼   **cup snipped fresh parsley**

In a medium bowl, stir together the beans, bell peppers, and onion.

In a small bowl, whisk together the remaining ingredients except the parsley. Pour over the bean mixture, tossing to coat. Stir in the parsley. Cover and refrigerate for 2 to 24 hours. Stir just before serving.

COOK'S TIP ON BALSAMIC VINEGAR
Balsamic vinegar is made from high-sugar grapes and aged in wooden barrels. The result is an intense, dark vinegar that is sweeter than most.

tabbouleh

SERVES 8
½ cup per serving

PREPARATION TIME
18 to 20 minutes

CHILLING TIME
2 to 24 hours

PER SERVING

Calories 121
Total Fat 3.5 g
    Saturated Fat 0.5 g
    Trans Fat 0.0 g
    Polyunsaturated Fat 0.5 g
    Monounsaturated Fat 2.5 g
Cholesterol 0 mg
Sodium 19 mg
Carbohydrates 21 g
    Fiber 4 g
    Sugars 8 g
Protein 3 g
Dietary Exchanges
    1 starch, ½ fruit, ½ fat

If you're looking for a traditional tabbouleh recipe, this isn't it. Currants, curry powder, cumin, and cinnamon make this jazzed-up version of tabbouleh different from the norm. Prepare Chickpea-Pistachio Dip (page 30) to continue the Middle Eastern theme of your meal.

SALAD

- ¾ cup uncooked fine bulgur
- ¾ cup boiling water
- 1 14.5-ounce can no-salt-added diced stewed tomatoes, undrained
- 1 cup snipped fresh parsley
- ½ cup snipped fresh mint
- ½ cup dried currants or raisins

DRESSING

- ¼ cup fat-free, low-sodium chicken broth
- ¼ cup fresh lemon juice
- 2 tablespoons olive oil (extra-virgin preferred)
- ½ teaspoon curry powder
- ½ teaspoon ground cumin
- ½ teaspoon ground cinnamon
- ½ teaspoon bottled minced garlic or 1 medium garlic clove, minced

In a small bowl, stir together the bulgur and water. Set aside.

In a large bowl, stir together the tomatoes with liquid, parsley, mint, and currants. Set aside.

In a separate small bowl, whisk together the dressing ingredients.

Stir the bulgur mixture into the tomato mixture. Pour the dressing over all, tossing to coat. Cover and refrigerate for 2 to 24 hours (the bulgur will absorb the liquid during refrigeration). Stir just before serving.

COOK'S TIP ON BULGUR
Fine bulgur, sometimes called number one grind, doesn't need any cooking; rather, a quick soak, as in this recipe, does the job. Look for it with other grains or pastas at your supermarket.

tuna salad bundles
WITH LEMON AND DILL

SERVES 4
2 bundles per serving

PREPARATION TIME
10 to 15 minutes

PER SERVING
Calories 131
Total Fat 1.5 g
  Saturated Fat 0.0 g
  Trans Fat 0.0 g
  Polyunsaturated Fat 0.0 g
  Monounsaturated Fat 0.0 g
Cholesterol 33 mg
Sodium 266 mg
Carbohydrates 7 g
  Fiber 2 g
  Sugars 4 g
Protein 26 g
Dietary Exchanges
  ½ other carbohydrate,
  3 very lean meat

These "salad sandwiches" use crisp romaine lettuce leaves to enfold a rich-tasting tuna and cottage cheese mixture seasoned with fresh dillweed and lots of lemon.

2   **5-ounce cans very low sodium white albacore tuna, packed in water, well drained and flaked**
1   **cup fat-free cottage cheese**
2   **to 3 medium green onions, sliced (about ¼ cup)**
2   **tablespoons snipped fresh dillweed or ¾ teaspoon dried, crumbled**
1   **teaspoon grated lemon zest**
1   **tablespoon fresh lemon juice**
¼   **teaspoon salt-free lemon pepper**
⅛   **teaspoon pepper**
8   **large romaine leaves**

In a medium bowl, stir together all the ingredients except the romaine. Cover and refrigerate until serving time or proceed as directed.

Spoon a generous ⅓ cup salad down the center of a romaine leaf, leaving about a half-inch uncovered at each end. Fold the sides of the leaf to the center and secure with a wooden toothpick if desired. Repeat with the remaining salad and romaine.

warm chicken and papaya salad

SERVES 4
1¼ cups per serving

PREPARATION TIME
20 minutes

COOKING TIME
3 to 5 minutes

PER SERVING
Calories 201
Total Fat 9.0 g
  Saturated Fat 1.5 g
  Trans Fat 0.0 g
  Polyunsaturated Fat 1.0 g
  Monounsaturated Fat 5.5 g
Cholesterol 54 mg
Sodium 123 mg
Carbohydrates 11 g
  Fiber 2 g
  Sugars 5 g
Protein 19 g
Dietary Exchanges
  ½ fruit, 2½ very lean meat,
  1 fat

Bite-size pieces of warm chicken top a vivid lettuce and radicchio salad studded with papaya cubes. Lime dressing adds a refreshingly tart note.

12   **ounces boneless, skinless chicken tenders, all visible fat discarded**

2   **tablespoons fresh lime juice and 2 tablespoons fresh lime juice, divided use**

4   **ounces lettuce, such as romaine or mixed salad greens, torn into bite-size pieces (about 4 cups)**

1   **ounce radicchio or red leaf lettuce, torn into bite-size pieces (about 1 cup)**

1   **medium papaya, peeled, seeded, and cubed (about 1½ cups)**

2   **to 3 medium green onions, sliced (about ¼ cup)**

2   **tablespoons olive oil (extra-virgin preferred)**

2   **tablespoons fat-free, low-sodium chicken broth**

½   **teaspoon Dijon mustard (lowest sodium available)**

½   **teaspoon bottled minced garlic or 1 medium garlic clove, minced**

⅛   **teaspoon pepper**
    Cooking spray

Put the chicken in a medium glass dish. Pour 2 tablespoons lime juice over the chicken, turning to coat. Set aside.

In a large bowl, toss together the lettuce, radicchio, papaya, and green onions. Set aside.

In a small bowl, whisk together the oil, broth, mustard, garlic, pepper, and remaining 2 tablespoons lime juice. Set aside.

Drain the chicken, discarding the marinade.

Lightly spray a large skillet with cooking spray. Heat over medium-high heat. Cook the chicken for 3 to 5 minutes, or until no longer pink in the center, turning once halfway through. Transfer to a cutting board. Cut into bite-size pieces.

Whisk the dressing and pour over the lettuce mixture, tossing to coat. Top with the chicken. Serve immediately for the best texture.

melon-chicken salad

SERVES 4
1¼ cups per serving

PREPARATION TIME
15 to 20 minutes

COOKING TIME
7 minutes

PER SERVING
Calories 219
Total Fat 6.0 g
  Saturated Fat 1.0 g
  Trans Fat 0.0 g
  Polyunsaturated Fat 3.0 g
  Monounsaturated Fat 1.5 g
Cholesterol 60 mg
Sodium 288 mg
Carbohydrates 21 g
  Fiber 3 g
  Sugars 17 g
Protein 21 g
Dietary Exchanges
1½ fruit, 2½ very lean meat,
½ fat

Cantaloupe and flavored yogurt set this chicken salad apart from the others.

12 **ounces boneless, skinless chicken breast tenders, all visible fat discarded**
1 **large or 2 small cantaloupes, cut into bite-size pieces**
2 **medium ribs of celery, sliced (about 1 cup)**
2 **tablespoons sliced green onions**
¼ **cup fat-free peach or vanilla yogurt**
¼ **cup light mayonnaise**
4 **large lettuce leaves, such as romaine or red leaf**

Pour water to a depth of 1 inch in a large skillet. Bring to a boil over high heat. Carefully add the chicken. Reduce the heat and simmer, covered, for 5 minutes, or until the chicken is no longer pink in the center. Drain well. Transfer to a cutting board. Set aside to cool slightly.

Meanwhile, in a large bowl, toss together the cantaloupe, celery, and green onions.

When the chicken is cool enough to handle, cut it into bite-size pieces. Add to the cantaloupe mixture, tossing to combine.

In a small bowl, whisk together the yogurt and mayonnaise. Pour over the salad, tossing to coat. Serve immediately, or cover and refrigerate until serving time. Just before serving, spoon the salad onto the lettuce leaves.

COOK'S TIP
Instead of poaching chicken and cutting cantaloupe into small pieces for this recipe, chop 2 cups of leftover chicken cooked without salt and buy 3 cups of chopped cantaloupe at the grocery store.

speedy taco salad

SERVES 4
2 cups per serving

PREPARATION TIME
10 minutes

COOKING TIME
8 minutes

PER SERVING

Calories 270
Total Fat 4.0 g
  Saturated Fat 2.0 g
  Trans Fat 0.0 g
  Polyunsaturated Fat 0.5 g
  Monounsaturated Fat 1.0 g
Cholesterol 62 mg
Sodium 295 mg
Carbohydrates 26 g
  Fiber 7 g
  Sugars 6 g
Protein 33 g
Dietary Exchanges
  1 starch, 2 vegetable,
  3½ very lean meat

For added crunch, serve this south-of-the-border salad with Homemade Corn Tortilla Chips (page 40) or commercial unsalted baked tortilla chips.

12 ounces ground skinless turkey breast or chicken breast
 1 15.5-ounce can no-salt-added red kidney beans, rinsed and drained
 1 14.5-ounce can no-salt-added diced tomatoes, drained
 1 4-ounce can chopped green chiles, drained
 1 tablespoon chili powder
 1 teaspoon ground cumin
 5 ounces lettuce, such as romaine or red leaf, torn into bite-size pieces (about 5 cups)
 ½ cup shredded low-fat Mexican blend cheese

In a large skillet, cook the turkey over medium-high heat for 5 minutes, or until browned on the outside and no longer pink in the center, stirring occasionally to turn and break up the turkey. Drain if needed.

Stir in the beans, tomatoes, chiles, chili powder, and cumin. Reduce the heat to medium and cook for 2 minutes, stirring frequently.

Put the lettuce on plates. Spoon the turkey mixture onto the lettuce. Sprinkle with the Mexican blend cheese. Serve immediately for the best texture.

pork and water chestnut salad
WITH CURRY DRESSING

SERVES 4
¾ cup per serving

PREPARATION TIME
10 to 12 minutes

COOKING TIME
6 minutes

COOLING TIME
5 minutes

PER SERVING
Calories 220
Total Fat 12.0 g
  Saturated Fat 2.0 g
  Trans Fat 0.0 g
  Polyunsaturated Fat 3.5 g
  Monounsaturated Fat 5.5 g
Cholesterol 34 mg
Sodium 241 mg
Carbohydrates 16 g
  Fiber 3 g
  Sugars 9 g
Protein 14 g
Dietary Exchanges
  1 other carbohydrate,
  2 lean meat, 1 fat

Three classic Asian ingredients—pork, water chestnuts, and curry powder—are key parts of this unique salad. It's sure to become a new lunchtime favorite!

SALAD
1 teaspoon canola or corn oil
8 ounces boneless center loin pork chops, all visible fat discarded, cut into ½-inch cubes
1 8-ounce can sliced water chestnuts, drained and chopped
⅓ cup sweetened dried cranberries
¼ cup finely chopped red onion
¼ cup chopped pecans, dry-roasted

DRESSING
2 tablespoons light mayonnaise
1 teaspoon curry powder
½ teaspoon ground cumin
¼ teaspoon ground nutmeg
¼ teaspoon salt
⅛ teaspoon crushed red pepper flakes (optional)

In a medium nonstick skillet, heat the oil over medium-high heat, swirling to coat the bottom. Cook the pork for 5 minutes, or until slightly pink in the center and light golden brown on the edges, stirring occasionally. Spoon in a single layer onto a large plate. Refrigerate for 5 minutes to cool quickly.

Meanwhile, in a medium bowl, stir together the remaining salad ingredients. Set aside.

In a small bowl, whisk together the dressing ingredients. Set aside.

Stir the cooled pork and any accumulated juices into the salad mixture. Pour in the dressing, tossing to combine.

layered two-bean salad

WITH CHEDDAR CHEESE

Whether you make this colorful salad as much as a day, or as little as an hour, in advance, it is a terrific find for easily fitting a meatless entrée into your menu plan.

3 ounces lettuce, such as romaine or red leaf, torn into bite-size pieces (about 3 cups)
1 15.5-ounce can no-salt-added red kidney beans, rinsed and drained
1 15.5-ounce can no-salt-added black beans, rinsed and drained
8 ounces presliced button mushrooms (about 2½ cups)
1 12-ounce can no-salt-added whole-kernel corn, drained
¼ cup chopped red onion
1 cup low-fat sour cream
¼ cup snipped fresh cilantro or parsley
2 tablespoons white wine vinegar
¼ teaspoon salt
⅛ teaspoon pepper
1 cup shredded fat-free Cheddar cheese

Put the lettuce in a large shallow glass bowl or baking dish. In the order listed, make one layer each of the following: kidney beans, black beans, mushrooms, corn, and onion.

In a small bowl, whisk together the remaining ingredients except the Cheddar. Spread over the salad, all the way to the sides. Sprinkle with the Cheddar. Cover and refrigerate for 1 to 24 hours before serving.

seafood

pasta-crusted fish

WITH MARINARA SAUCE

SERVES 4
3 ounces fish and
¼ cup sauce
per serving

PREPARATION TIME
8 to 10 minutes

COOKING TIME
8 to 10 minutes

PER SERVING
Calories 212
Total Fat 2.0 g
  Saturated Fat 0.0 g
  Trans Fat 0.0 g
  Polyunsaturated Fat 0.0 g
  Monounsaturated Fat 0.0 g
Cholesterol 43 mg
Sodium 318 mg
Carbohydrates 25 g
  Fiber 2 g
  Sugars 3 g
Protein 23 g
Dietary Exchanges
  1½ starch, 1 vegetable,
  3 very lean meat

For an unusual coating, press bits of uncooked fresh angel hair pasta onto fish fillets. While they bake, the pasta forms a crisp coating.

Cooking spray

1 cup finely chopped uncooked fresh angel hair pasta

4 mild white fish fillets (about 4 ounces each), rinsed and patted dry

¼ teaspoon dried dillweed, crumbled

Pepper to taste

1 cup marinara sauce (lowest sodium available)

Preheat the oven to 450°F. Lightly spray a baking sheet with cooking spray.

Put the pasta in a medium shallow dish. Press one side of one piece of fish into the pasta to coat well. Transfer with the pasta side up to the baking sheet. Repeat with the remaining pasta and fish, arranging the fish in a single layer on the baking sheet. Sprinkle the fish with the dillweed and pepper. Lightly spray with cooking spray.

Bake for 8 to 10 minutes, or until the fish flakes easily when tested with a fork.

Meanwhile, in a small saucepan, cook the marinara sauce over medium-low heat for 5 minutes, or until heated through. Spoon over the fish.

COOK'S TIP ON MILD WHITE FISH
A number of factors may affect your choice of fish for this and other recipes that call for mild white fish. Taste preference, availability, freshness, price, and avoidance of what is currently being overharvested are some of the main things to consider. Fortunately, many mild white fish are interchangeable, with only minor adjustments needed in cooking time if you choose fillets or steaks much thicker or much thinner than called for. Some of the many examples of mild white fish are cod, grouper, haddock, mahimahi, sea bass, scrod, sole, and tilapia.

pecan-coated fillets

WITH CORN RELISH

SERVES 4
3 ounces fish and
⅓ cup relish
per serving

PREPARATION TIME
10 to 12 minutes

COOKING TIME
10 to 15 minutes

PER SERVING
Calories 215
Total Fat 9.5 g
  Saturated Fat 1.0 g
  Trans Fat 0.0 g
  Polyunsaturated Fat 3.5 g
  Monounsaturated Fat 4.5 g
Cholesterol 46 mg
Sodium 202 mg
Carbohydrates 14 g
  Fiber 2 g
  Sugars 3 g
Protein 20 g
Dietary Exchanges
  1 starch, 3 lean meat

Pecans provide a delightful crunch to these mild fish fillets, which bake while the flavors of the relish ingredients are blending.

Cooking spray
1 cup drained canned no-salt-added whole-kernel corn
½ medium green bell pepper, chopped
¼ cup chopped red onion
2 tablespoons snipped fresh cilantro or parsley
2 tablespoons fresh lime juice
½ teaspoon bottled minced garlic or 1 medium garlic clove, minced
⅛ teaspoon cayenne
⅛ teaspoon salt
4 mild white fish fillets (about 4 ounces each), rinsed and patted dry
2 tablespoons light mayonnaise
Pepper to taste
⅓ cup chopped pecans, dry-roasted

Preheat the oven to 450°F. Using cooking spray, lightly spray a shallow glass baking dish large enough to hold the fish in a single layer.

In a medium bowl, stir together the corn, bell pepper, onion, cilantro, lime juice, garlic, cayenne, and salt. Set aside.

Put the fish in the baking dish, tucking the thin edges under for even cooking. Lightly brush the top of the fish with the mayonnaise. Sprinkle with the pepper and pecans.

Bake for 10 to 15 minutes, or until the fish flakes easily when tested with a fork. Serve with the relish.

fish and fettuccine

SERVES 4
one 4½-inch square
per serving

PREPARATION TIME
10 minutes

COOKING TIME
35 to 40 minutes

STANDING TIME
5 minutes

PER SERVING
Calories 318
Total Fat 3.5 g
    Saturated Fat 1.5 g
    Trans Fat 0.0 g
    Polyunsaturated Fat 0.5 g
    Monounsaturated Fat 0.5 g
Cholesterol 95 mg
Sodium 327 mg
Carbohydrates 41 g
    Fiber 3 g
    Sugars 5 g
Protein 29 g
Dietary Exchanges
    2 starch, 2 vegetable,
    3 very lean meat

With its layers of tomatoes, spinach fettuccine, summer squash, fish, and seasonings, this pasta-generous casserole is an easy meal-in-one.

1 **14.5-ounce can no-salt-added diced stewed tomatoes, undrained**

4 **mild white fish fillets (about 4 ounces each), rinsed and patted dry**

1 **9-ounce package uncooked fresh spinach fettuccine, coarsely chopped**

2 **small yellow summer squash, sliced**

2 **tablespoons chopped shallots**

2 **tablespoons snipped fresh basil or 1 teaspoon dried, crumbled**

2 **tablespoons snipped fresh oregano or 1 teaspoon dried, crumbled**

¼ **teaspoon salt**

2 **tablespoons shredded or grated Parmesan or Romano cheese**

Preheat the oven to 425°F.

Pour the tomatoes with liquid into a 9-inch square glass baking dish. Make one layer each of the fish, pasta, summer squash, shallots, basil, and oregano. Sprinkle with the salt.

Bake, tightly covered, for 35 to 40 minutes, or until the fish flakes easily when tested with a fork. Remove from the oven. Sprinkle with the Parmesan. Let stand, covered, for 5 minutes before serving.

creole catfish

SERVES 4
3 ounces fish and ⅓ cup sauce per serving

PREPARATION TIME
12 to 15 minutes

COOKING TIME
17 minutes

PER SERVING
Calories 151
Total Fat 4.5 g
   Saturated Fat 1.0 g
   Trans Fat 0.0 g
   Polyunsaturated Fat 1.0 g
   Monounsaturated Fat 2.0 g
Cholesterol 66 mg
Sodium 211 mg
Carbohydrates 7 g
   Fiber 2 g
   Sugars 4 g
Protein 20 g
Dietary Exchanges
   1 vegetable, 3 lean meat

Flavored with paprika and two kinds of pepper, this is a fish dish with a kick. Serve it with brown rice to soak up all the delicious sauce.

Cooking spray
2 teaspoons paprika
¼ teaspoon salt
¼ teaspoon pepper
Pinch of cayenne

SAUCE
1 teaspoon olive oil
½ medium rib of celery, diced
¼ medium red bell pepper, diced
¼ cup diced onion
½ teaspoon bottled minced garlic or 1 medium garlic clove, minced
1 14.5-ounce can no-salt-added diced tomatoes, undrained

2 catfish or other mild white fish fillets (about 8 ounces each), rinsed and patted dry

Preheat the broiler. Line a baking sheet with aluminum foil. Lightly spray the foil with cooking spray. Set aside.

In a small dish, stir together the paprika, salt, pepper, and cayenne. Set aside.

In a medium skillet, heat the oil over medium-high heat, swirling to coat the bottom. Cook the celery, bell pepper, onion, and garlic for 3 minutes, stirring frequently.

Stir in the tomatoes with liquid. Using a potato masher, mash the vegetables to make the sauce somewhat smoother.

Stir in 1½ teaspoons of the paprika mixture, setting the remaining mixture aside. Bring the sauce to a boil. Reduce the heat and simmer for 10 minutes, or until the vegetables are tender and the sauce is thickened.

Meanwhile, sprinkle the fish on both sides with the remaining 1 teaspoon paprika mixture. Using your fingertips, gently press the seasonings so they adhere to the fish. Transfer to the baking sheet.

Broil on one side about 4 inches from the heat for 8 minutes, or until the fish flakes easily when tested with a fork. Cut each fillet in half. Serve topped with the sauce.

crunchy fish nuggets
WITH LEMON TARTAR SAUCE

The panko coating makes these bite-size pieces of fish crunchy on the outside and keeps them wonderfully moist on the inside.

　　Cooking spray
2　large egg whites
2　tablespoons fat-free milk
¼　cup whole-wheat panko (Japanese bread crumbs)
¼　cup shredded or grated Parmesan cheese
½　teaspoon paprika
1　pound halibut steaks or fillets, rinsed and patted dry, cut into 24 bite-size pieces

SAUCE
½　cup light mayonnaise
2　tablespoons finely chopped dill pickle
1　teaspoon grated lemon zest
1　teaspoon fresh lemon juice

Preheat the oven to 450°F. Lightly spray a large baking sheet with cooking spray. Set aside.

　　In a medium shallow dish, whisk together the egg whites and milk.

　　In a separate medium shallow dish, stir together the panko, Parmesan, and paprika.

　　Put the dishes and baking sheet in a row, assembly-line fashion. Working in batches and using a slotted spoon, put the fish in the egg white mixture, turning to coat and letting any excess drip off. Transfer to the panko mixture, turning to coat well and gently shaking off any excess. Transfer to the baking sheet, arranging the fish in a single layer.

　　Bake for 5 minutes, or until the fish flakes easily when tested with a fork.

　　Meanwhile, in a small bowl, stir together the tartar sauce ingredients. Serve with the fish.

broiled halibut

WITH CHUNKY TOMATO-CREAM SAUCE

The versatile tomato and sour cream sauce that tops the halibut can double as an easy pasta sauce.

   Cooking spray
2 halibut steaks (about 8 ounces each), about 1 inch thick, rinsed and patted dry
1 teaspoon olive oil
   Pepper to taste

SAUCE

1 14.5-ounce can no-salt-added stewed tomatoes, chopped, undrained
½ teaspoon bottled minced garlic or 1 medium garlic clove, minced
¼ cup fat-free sour cream
1 tablespoon all-purpose flour
1 teaspoon dried Italian seasoning, crumbled
¼ teaspoon salt

Preheat the broiler. Lightly spray a broiler pan and rack with cooking spray.

Put the fish on the rack. Lightly brush the top of the fish with the oil. Sprinkle with the pepper.

Broil about 4 inches from the heat for 5 minutes. Turn over. Broil for 3 to 7 minutes, or until the fish flakes easily when tested with a fork. Cut each fish steak in half.

Meanwhile, in a medium saucepan, stir together the tomatoes with liquid and the garlic. Cook over medium-high heat for 5 minutes, or until bubbly.

In a small bowl, whisk together the sour cream, flour, Italian seasoning, and salt. Stir into the tomato mixture. Cook for 4 to 5 minutes, or until bubbly and thickened to the desired consistency, whisking constantly.

Serve the fish with the seasoned side up. Spoon the sauce over the fish.

halibut

WITH GREEN TEA GLAZE

SERVES 4
3 ounces fish per serving

PREPARATION TIME
10 minutes

COOKING TIME
21 to 22 minutes

PER SERVING
Calories 162
Total Fat 2.5 g
  Saturated Fat 0.5 g
  Trans Fat 0.0 g
  Polyunsaturated Fat 1.0 g
  Monounsaturated Fat 1.0 g
Cholesterol 36 mg
Sodium 65 mg
Carbohydrates 10 g
  Fiber 0 g
  Sugars 9 g
Protein 24 g
Dietary Exchanges
  ½ other carbohydrate,
  3 very lean meat

A reduction of green tea, honey, and lime juice produces an intensely flavored glaze that makes an excellent counterpoint to the mild flavor of halibut.

1   **cup unsweetened green tea**
2   **tablespoons honey**
2   **tablespoons fresh lime juice**
¼   **cup loosely packed fresh mint**
¼   **teaspoon crushed red pepper flakes**
4   **halibut fillets (about 4 ounces each), rinsed and patted dry**
1   **medium lime, cut into 4 wedges**

Preheat the broiler.

In a medium saucepan, stir together the tea, honey, and lime juice. Bring to a boil over high heat. Boil for 8 minutes, or until the mixture is syrupy and reduced to about ¼ cup. Remove from the heat.

Stir in the mint and red pepper flakes. Let steep for 1 minute. Discard the mint.

Place the fish on a rimmed baking sheet. Drizzle 1 tablespoon of the glaze over the top of the fish. Set the remaining glaze aside.

Broil the fish 4 to 6 inches from the heat for 4 minutes. Turn over. Drizzle 1 tablespoon of the glaze over the fish. Set the remaining glaze aside. Broil for 4 to 5 minutes, or until the fish flakes easily when tested with a fork.

Transfer the fish to plates. Drizzle the remaining glaze over the fish. Serve with the lime wedges to squeeze over the fish.

grilled salmon
WITH MANGO-LIME CREAM SAUCE

This refreshing yet rich-tasting sauce adds an unusual flavor kick to simple grilled salmon.

  Cooking spray
⅛ teaspoon salt
⅛ teaspoon pepper (white preferred)
 4 salmon fillets (about 4 ounces each), rinsed and patted dry

SAUCE
⅓ cup coarsely chopped bottled mango, 1 tablespoon juice reserved
¼ cup fat-free sour cream
½ teaspoon grated lime zest
1 teaspoon fresh lime juice

Lightly spray the grill rack with cooking spray. Preheat the grill on medium high.

Sprinkle the salt and pepper over one side of the salmon. Using your fingertips, gently press so they adhere to the fish.

Grill with the seasoned side down for 5 minutes. Turn over. Grill for 2 to 3 minutes, or to the desired doneness.

Meanwhile, in a small bowl, whisk together all the sauce ingredients. Serve at room temperature or cover and refrigerate until serving time. Spoon over the fish.

COOK'S TIP ON MANGOES
Check the refrigerated area of the produce section for sliced mangoes in jars. They save on time and are less messy.

jerked salmon

WITH RASPBERRY-MINT SALSA

SERVES 4
3 ounces fish and
⅓ cup salsa
per serving

PREPARATION TIME
15 minutes

COOKING TIME
7 to 8 minutes

PER SERVING
Calories 181
Total Fat 4.5 g
  Saturated Fat 0.5 g
  Trans Fat 0.0 g
  Polyunsaturated Fat 2.0 g
  Monounsaturated Fat 1.0 g
Cholesterol 65 mg
Sodium 231 mg
Carbohydrates 9 g
  Fiber 3 g
  Sugars 5 g
Protein 25 g
Dietary Exchanges
  ½ fruit, 3 lean meat

The minty cool fruit salsa balances out the heat of the peppery grilled salmon in this pretty entrée.

Cooking spray

SALSA

1⅓ cups fresh or frozen unsweetened raspberries, thawed if frozen

¼ cup finely chopped red onion

2 tablespoons snipped fresh mint

1½ teaspoons sugar

½ teaspoon grated orange zest

2 tablespoons fresh orange juice

1 teaspoon salt-free jerk seasoning blend

½ teaspoon pepper (coarsely ground preferred)

¼ teaspoon salt

4 salmon fillets with skin (about 5 ounces each), rinsed and patted dry

Lightly spray the grill rack with cooking spray. Preheat the grill on medium.

Meanwhile, in a small bowl, stir together the salsa ingredients. Set aside.

In a separate small bowl, stir together the seasoning blend, pepper, and salt. Sprinkle over the top and sides of the fish. Using your fingertips, gently press the seasonings so they adhere to the fish.

Grill the fish with the skin side down for 5 minutes. Turn over. Grill for 2 to 3 minutes, or until cooked to the desired doneness. Serve with the salsa.

COOK'S TIP ON JERK SEASONING

To make your own salt-free jerk seasoning, in a small bowl, stir together ½ teaspoon ground cumin, ¼ teaspoon ground allspice, ¼ teaspoon ground cinnamon, and ⅛ to ¼ teaspoon cayenne.

COOK'S TIP ON SALSAS

Add some zip to your salsas, whether they're fruit- or veggie-based, by substituting fresh mint for the usual cilantro or parsley. Just be sure to make the salsa at least 10 minutes in advance so the flavors have time to blend.

spinach-topped salmon

SERVES 4
3 ounces fish and
¼ cup spinach mixture
per serving

PREPARATION TIME
8 minutes

COOKING TIME
15 to 18 minutes

PER SERVING
Calories 193
Total Fat 5.0 g
  Saturated Fat 1.0 g
  Trans Fat 0.0 g
  Polyunsaturated Fat 1.5 g
  Monounsaturated Fat 1.5 g
Cholesterol 67 mg
Sodium 166 mg
Carbohydrates 3 g
  Fiber 2 g
  Sugars 1 g
Protein 28 g
Dietary Exchanges
  3 lean meat

A bay leaf and a bit of nutmeg add subtle but interesting flavor to this attractive dish, with contrasting colors provided by the salmon, spinach, and mozzarella cheese.

Cooking spray

1½ cups water

½ cup dry white wine (regular or nonalcoholic) or water

2 medium green onions, sliced

1 medium dried bay leaf

4 salmon fillets (about 4 ounces each), rinsed and patted dry

5 ounces frozen chopped spinach

⅛ teaspoon ground nutmeg

¼ cup shredded low-fat mozzarella cheese

Pepper to taste

1 medium lemon, thinly sliced (optional)

Preheat the broiler. Lightly spray the broiler pan and rack with cooking spray. Set aside.

In a large skillet, bring the water, wine, green onions, and bay leaf just to a boil over high heat. Using a large spatula, carefully add each piece of fish. Return to a boil. Reduce the heat and simmer, covered, for 8 to 10 minutes, or until the fish is the desired doneness. Transfer the fish to the broiler rack. Discard the cooking liquid. Pat the fish dry with paper towels.

Meanwhile, prepare the spinach using the package directions. Drain well, squeezing out the moisture. Stir in the nutmeg. Spread over the fish.

Sprinkle the mozzarella and pepper over the spinach.

Broil about 4 inches from the heat for 1 to 2 minutes, or until the mozzarella melts. Garnish the fish with the lemon.

COOK'S TIP

To use half of a 10-ounce package of frozen spinach for this recipe, here's what to do: Place the unwrapped block of spinach on a microwaveable plate and cook on 30 percent power (medium low) for 2 minutes, or until the spinach is just soft enough to cut through with a sharp knife. Use half the package as directed in the recipe. Rewrap and return the remaining half to the freezer.

salmon and brown rice bake

SERVES 4
1 cup per serving

PREPARATION TIME
5 to 7 minutes

COOKING TIME
35 minutes

PER SERVING
Calories 186
Total Fat 3.0 g
 Saturated Fat 1.0 g
 Trans Fat 0.0 g
 Polyunsaturated Fat 1.0 g
 Monounsaturated Fat 0.5 g
Cholesterol 14 mg
Sodium 303 mg
Carbohydrates 30 g
 Fiber 3 g
 Sugars 3 g
Protein 12 g
Dietary Exchanges
 2 starch, 1 very lean meat

This recipe may remind you of that traditional favorite, tuna-noodle casserole. For a change of pace, we use salmon instead of tuna and brown rice instead of noodles.

10 **ounces frozen whole-kernel corn**
¾ **cup uncooked instant brown rice**
1 **6-ounce vacuum-sealed pouch boneless, skinless pink salmon, flaked**
⅔ **cup water**
2 **tablespoons sliced green onions**
½ **teaspoon very low sodium chicken bouillon granules**
¼ **teaspoon dried dillweed, crumbled**
⅛ **teaspoon salt**
¼ **cup shredded low-fat Cheddar cheese**

Preheat the oven to 375°F.

In a 1½-quart glass casserole dish, stir together all the ingredients except the Cheddar.

Bake, covered, for 30 minutes, or until the rice is tender. Sprinkle with the Cheddar. Bake, uncovered, for 5 minutes, or until the Cheddar is melted.

spicy sole and tomatoes

SERVES 4
3 ounces fish per serving

PREPARATION TIME
8 minutes

COOKING TIME
9 to 11 minutes

PER SERVING

Calories 136
Total Fat 1.5 g
  Saturated Fat 0.5 g
  Trans Fat 0.0 g
  Polyunsaturated Fat 0.5 g
  Monounsaturated Fat 0.5 g
Cholesterol 54 mg
Sodium 127 mg
Carbohydrates 7 g
  Fiber 1 g
  Sugars 4 g
Protein 22 g
Dietary Exchanges
  1 vegetable, 3 very lean
  meat

Serve this snappy fish dish with corn on the cob and a salad of mixed baby greens with carrots, bell pepper, and cucumber.

Cooking spray
½ cup chopped onion
½ teaspoon bottled minced garlic or 1 medium garlic clove, minced
1 14.5-ounce can no-salt-added diced tomatoes, undrained
1 teaspoon capers, drained
4 peppercorns
4 to 6 dashes red hot-pepper sauce, or to taste
4 sole or other mild white fish fillets (about 4 ounces each), rinsed and patted dry

Lightly spray a large skillet with cooking spray. Cook the onion and garlic over medium-high heat for 3 minutes, or until the onion is soft, stirring frequently.

Stir in the remaining ingredients except the fish. Bring to a boil.

Place the fish on the tomato mixture. Return to a boil. Reduce the heat and simmer, covered, for 4 to 6 minutes, or until the fish flakes easily when tested with a fork. Discard the peppercorns before serving the fish.

baked tilapia
WITH PINEAPPLE REDUCTION

SERVES 4
3 ounces fish and
1 tablespoon sauce
per serving

PREPARATION TIME
8 minutes

COOKING TIME
8 minutes

PER SERVING
Calories 183
Total Fat 5.5 g
  Saturated Fat 1.0 g
  Trans Fat 0.0 g
  Polyunsaturated Fat 1.5 g
  Monounsaturated Fat 3.0 g
Cholesterol 57 mg
Sodium 256 mg
Carbohydrates 9 g
  Fiber 0 g
  Sugars 7 g
Protein 23 g
Dietary Exchanges
  ½ fruit, 3 lean meat

A simple fruit juice reduction, mixed with soy sauce and curry powder, provides an abundance of flavor for these baked fish fillets.

  Cooking spray
4 tilapia or other mild white fish fillets (about 4 ounces each), rinsed and patted dry
1 tablespoon canola or corn oil
¼ teaspoon pepper
⅛ teaspoon cayenne (optional)

SAUCE
2 tablespoons soy sauce (lowest sodium available)
1 tablespoon cider vinegar
2 teaspoons sugar
1½ teaspoons cornstarch
½ teaspoon curry powder
⅛ teaspoon crushed red pepper flakes (optional)
¾ cup pineapple juice

Preheat the oven to 450°F. Line a baking sheet with aluminum foil. Lightly spray the foil with cooking spray.

Place the fish on the baking sheet. Brush the top of the fish with the oil. Sprinkle the top with the pepper and cayenne. Using your fingertips, gently press the seasonings so they adhere to the fish.

Bake for 8 minutes, or until the fish flakes easily when tested with a fork.

Meanwhile, in small bowl, whisk together the sauce ingredients except the pineapple juice until the cornstarch is dissolved. Set aside.

In a large saucepan, bring the pineapple juice to a boil over high heat. Boil for 2 to 3 minutes, or until reduced to ⅓ cup. Whisk the soy sauce mixture into the pineapple juice. Reduce the heat to medium high and cook for 1 minute, or until the mixture is slightly thickened, whisking frequently. Serve over the fish.

COOK'S TIP ON REDUCTIONS
When working with reductions, it's best to use a large saucepan or skillet, even with small amounts of liquid, to keep spattering to a minimum.

tex-mex tilapia packets

SERVES 4
3 ounces fish per serving

PREPARATION TIME
15 minutes

COOKING TIME
10 to 12 minutes

PER SERVING
Calories 189
Total Fat 5.5 g
  Saturated Fat 1.5 g
  Trans Fat 0.0 g
  Polyunsaturated Fat 1.0 g
  Monounsaturated Fat 3.0 g
Cholesterol 62 mg
Sodium 289 mg
Carbohydrates 11 g
  Fiber 1 g
  Sugars 4 g
Protein 25 g
Dietary Exchanges
  ½ other carbohydrate,
  3 lean meat

Baking these tilapia fillets in aluminum foil packets seals in their juices and seasonings, keeping the fish extra-moist and flavorful.

Cooking spray
1 **medium lemon or lime, cut into 8 slices, and 1 medium lemon or lime, cut into 4 wedges, divided use**
4 **tilapia or other mild white fish fillets (about 4 ounces each), rinsed and patted dry**
¼ **cup mild picante sauce and ¼ cup mild picante sauce (lowest sodium available), divided use**
4 **medium green onions, chopped**
2 **medium fresh jalapeños, seeds and ribs discarded, finely chopped**
1 **tablespoon olive oil (extra-virgin preferred)**
½ **cup fat-free sour cream**
¼ **teaspoon pepper (coarsely ground preferred)**

Preheat the oven to 425°F. Cut eight 12-inch square pieces of aluminum foil. Lightly spray one side of each with cooking spray.

Place 2 lemon slices in the center of the sprayed side of four pieces of foil. Place the fish on the lemon slices. Top each serving with about 1 tablespoon picante sauce. Sprinkle with the green onions and jalapeños. Put one of the remaining pieces of foil with the sprayed side down over each serving. Fold the edges together several times to seal each packet securely so the juices don't leak out. Transfer to a large baking sheet.

Bake for 10 minutes. Using the tines of a fork, carefully open one of the packets away from you (to prevent steam burns). If the fish flakes easily when tested with the fork, it is done, and you can then carefully open the remaining packets. If the fish in the opened packet isn't cooked enough, reseal the packet and continue baking all the packets for about 2 minutes.

Meanwhile, in a small bowl, stir together the oil and remaining ¼ cup picante sauce. Spoon 1 tablespoon of the mixture over each serving. Top each with 2 table-spoons sour cream. Sprinkle with the pepper. Serve the remaining lemon wedges to squeeze over the fish.

broiled tilapia

WITH BLACK BEAN SALSA

SERVES 4
3 ounces fish and
⅓ cup salsa per serving

PREPARATION TIME
10 to 12 minutes

COOKING TIME
7 to 9 minutes

PER SERVING
Calories 226
Total Fat 2.0 g
  Saturated Fat 1.0 g
  Trans Fat 0.0 g
  Polyunsaturated Fat 0.5 g
  Monounsaturated Fat 0.5 g
Cholesterol 57 mg
Sodium 231 mg
Carbohydrates 22 g
  Fiber 6 g
  Sugars 6 g
Protein 29 g
Dietary Exchanges
  1 starch, 1 vegetable,
  3½ very lean meat

The hearty salsa that tops these broiled tilapia fillets packs a lot of Tex-Mex punch.

Cooking spray
4 tilapia or other mild white fish fillets (about 4 ounces each), rinsed and patted dry
1 medium lime, halved crosswise, divided use
1 15.5-ounce can no-salt-added black beans, about 1 inch of liquid drained off
4 medium green onions, sliced
1 medium rib of celery, chopped
1 medium carrot, chopped
1 teaspoon ground cumin
½ teaspoon bottled minced garlic or 1 medium garlic clove, minced
¼ teaspoon minced fresh jalapeño, seeds and ribs discarded
¼ cup snipped fresh cilantro or parsley (optional)
¼ teaspoon salt

Preheat the broiler. Lightly spray a broiler pan and rack with cooking spray.

Put the fish on the rack. Squeeze the juice from one lime half over the fish.

Broil the fish about 4 inches from the heat for 4 minutes. Turn over. Squeeze the juice from the remaining lime half over the fish. Broil for 2 to 4 minutes, or until the fish flakes easily when tested with a fork.

Meanwhile, in a medium saucepan, cook the beans and remaining liquid, green onions, celery, carrot, cumin, garlic, and jalapeño over medium-low heat for 6 to 8 minutes, or until the fish is done, stirring occasionally. Stir in the cilantro and salt. Spoon over the fish.

COOK'S TIP
You can make and refrigerate the salsa without the cilantro and salt up to 24 hours in advance. To serve, bring the salsa to room temperature and add the cilantro and salt, or reheat the salsa over low heat, then stir them in.

grilled trout

WITH CREAMY CAPER-DILL SAUCE

SERVES 4
3 ounces fish and
2 tablespoons sauce
per serving

PREPARATION TIME
8 to 10 minutes

COOKING TIME
6 to 8 minutes

PER SERVING
Calories 182
Total Fat 7.5 g
　Saturated Fat 1.5 g
　Trans Fat 0.0 g
　Polyunsaturated Fat 2.0 g
　Monounsaturated Fat 3.5 g
Cholesterol 67 mg
Sodium 319 mg
Carbohydrates 2 g
　Fiber 0 g
　Sugars 1 g
Protein 26 g
Dietary Exchanges
　3 lean meat

Greek yogurt teams with capers, herbs, and garlic to create a rich-tasting sauce for peppery grilled trout fillets.

　　Cooking spray
SAUCE
　½　cup fat-free Greek yogurt
　2　tablespoons capers, drained and chopped
　1½　teaspoons snipped fresh dillweed or ½ teaspoon dried, crumbled
　½　teaspoon bottled minced garlic or 1 medium garlic clove, minced
　¾　teaspoon snipped fresh oregano or ¼ teaspoon dried, crumbled
　⅛　teaspoon salt

　4　trout fillets (about 4 ounces each), rinsed and patted dry
　1　tablespoon olive oil
　½　teaspoon pepper (coarsely ground preferred)
　⅛　teaspoon salt

Lightly spray the grill rack with cooking spray. Preheat the grill on medium.

　In a small bowl, whisk together the sauce ingredients. Set aside.

　Brush both sides of the fish with the oil. Sprinkle with the pepper and remaining ⅛ teaspoon salt.

　Grill for 3 minutes. Carefully turn over. Grill for 3 to 5 minutes, or until the fish flakes easily when tested with a fork. Serve with the sauce.

COOK'S TIP ON GRILLING FISH FILLETS
Some fish fillets are rather fragile, so you'll need to handle them with care when turning them on the grill. If you have a perforated flat grilling pan or a grilling basket for fish, it will help you keep the fillets intact.

COOK'S TIP ON CAPERS
Even if you use small capers, chop them to spread the flavor through the dish.

smoky trout

WITH CITRUS TOPPING

SERVES 4
3 ounces fish and
2 tablespoons topping
per serving

PREPARATION TIME
8 minutes

COOKING TIME
6 to 8 minutes

MICROWAVE TIME
15 seconds

PER SERVING

Calories 173
Total Fat 7.5 g
  Saturated Fat 2.0 g
  Trans Fat 0.0 g
  Polyunsaturated Fat 2.5 g
  Monounsaturated Fat 3.0 g
Cholesterol 67 mg
Sodium 334 mg
Carbohydrates 0 g
  Fiber 0 g
  Sugars 0 g
Protein 23 g
Dietary Exchanges
  3 lean meat

Ever so delicious and ever so simple, this dish features a three-ingredient topping that takes only seconds to prepare. Grill asparagus spears to serve on the side.

Cooking spray
1 teaspoon salt-free grilling seasoning blend
½ teaspoon smoked paprika
¼ teaspoon salt
4 trout fillets (about 4 ounces each), rinsed and patted dry

TOPPING
3 tablespoons light tub margarine
1½ teaspoons Louisiana hot sauce
½ teaspoon grated orange zest

Lightly spray the grill rack with cooking spray. Preheat the grill on medium.

In a small bowl, stir together the seasoning blend, paprika, and salt.

Lightly spray the fish on both sides with cooking spray. Sprinkle all over with the seasoning blend mixture. Using your fingertips, gently press the seasonings so they adhere to the fish.

Grill for 3 minutes. Carefully turn over. Grill for 3 to 5 minutes, or until the fish flakes easily when tested with a fork.

Meanwhile, in a small microwaveable bowl, microwave the margarine on 100 percent power (high) for 15 seconds, or until just melted. Remove from the microwave. Whisk in the hot sauce and orange zest. Spoon over the fish.

spice-baked trout fillets

SERVES 4
3 ounces fish per serving

PREPARATION TIME
8 minutes

COOKING TIME
8 minutes

PER SERVING
Calories 172
Total Fat 7.5 g
  Saturated Fat 1.0 g
  Trans Fat 0.0 g
  Polyunsaturated Fat 2.5 g
  Monounsaturated Fat 3.5 g
Cholesterol 67 mg
Sodium 181 mg
Carbohydrates 1 g
  Fiber 0 g
  Sugars 1 g
Protein 23 g
Dietary Exchanges
  3 lean meat

Brush the fish with oil, sprinkle with seasonings, and bake—that's all you need to do to get these fillets ready to serve. The bonus is that the mixture makes its own sweet, smoky sauce as it bakes. Citrus Kale with Dried Cranberries (page 215) makes a good accompaniment.

  Cooking spray
4 trout fillets (about 4 ounces each), rinsed and patted dry
1 tablespoon canola or corn oil
1 teaspoon smoked paprika
¾ teaspoon sugar
½ teaspoon ground cumin
¼ teaspoon salt
⅛ teaspoon ground allspice
⅛ teaspoon ground cinnamon
  Dash of cayenne

Preheat the oven to 450°F. Line a baking sheet with aluminum foil. Lightly spray the foil with cooking spray.

Place the fish on the baking sheet. Brush the top of the fish with the oil.

In a small bowl, stir together the remaining ingredients. Sprinkle over the top of the fish.

Bake for 8 minutes, or until the fish flakes easily when tested with a fork.

tuna

WITH GINGER BOK CHOY

SERVES 4
3 ounces fish and
½ cup bok choy
per serving

PREPARATION TIME
10 to 12 minutes

COOKING TIME
10 minutes

PER SERVING
Calories 186
Total Fat 5.5 g
 Saturated Fat 0.5 g
 Trans Fat 0.0 g
 Polyunsaturated Fat 2.0 g
 Monounsaturated Fat 2.0 g
Cholesterol 51 mg
Sodium 316 mg
Carbohydrates 5 g
 Fiber 2 g
 Sugars 3 g
Protein 30 g
Dietary Exchanges
 1 vegetable, 3 lean meat

Ginger and garlic give the bok choy an incredible flavor that accents the simply prepared tuna in this dish.

2 **tuna steaks (about 8 ounces each), cut about ½ inch thick, rinsed and patted dry, halved**
⅛ **teaspoon salt**
⅛ **teaspoon pepper**
1 **teaspoon canola or corn oil and 1 teaspoon canola or corn oil, divided use**
2 **teaspoons minced peeled gingerroot**
½ **teaspoon bottled minced garlic or 1 medium garlic clove, minced**
1 **small head of bok choy or ½ medium head of napa cabbage, thinly sliced (about 8 cups)**
2 **teaspoons soy sauce (lowest sodium available)**
1¼ **teaspoons toasted sesame oil**

Sprinkle both sides of the fish with the salt and pepper. Using your fingertips, gently press the seasonings so they adhere to the fish.

In a large nonstick skillet, heat 1 teaspoon canola oil over medium-high heat, swirling to coat the bottom. Cook the fish for 2 minutes on each side, or to the desired doneness. Transfer to a plate. Cover to keep warm.

In the same skillet, heat the remaining 1 teaspoon canola oil, swirling to coat the bottom. Cook the gingerroot and garlic for 30 seconds, or until fragrant, stirring constantly.

Stir in the bok choy. Cook for 3 minutes, or until just wilted, stirring occasionally.

Stir in the soy sauce. Spoon the bok choy onto plates. Top with the fish. Drizzle with the sesame oil.

pan-seared tuna

WITH MANDARIN ORANGE PICO DE GALLO

SERVES 4
3 ounces fish and
⅓ cup pico de gallo
per serving

PREPARATION TIME
10 minutes

COOKING TIME
11 minutes

PER SERVING
Calories 185
Total Fat 3.0 g
　Saturated Fat 0.5 g
　Trans Fat 0.0 g
　Polyunsaturated Fat 0.5 g
　Monounsaturated Fat 1.5 g
Cholesterol 51 mg
Sodium 49 mg
Carbohydrates 11 g
　Fiber 2 g
　Sugars 8 g
Protein 28 g
Dietary Exchanges
　½ fruit, 1 vegetable,
　3 very lean meat

Not too spicy and not too sweet, this fruit-based pico de gallo is just right! Try it with mild tuna steaks, as here, or with other fish or chicken.

Cooking spray

PICO DE GALLO
- ½ **cup chopped red or yellow onion**
- ½ **teaspoon bottled minced garlic or 1 medium garlic clove, minced**
- 1 **tablespoon balsamic vinegar or red wine vinegar**
- 1 **teaspoon firmly packed light brown sugar**
- ⅛ **to ¼ teaspoon crushed red pepper flakes**
- 1 **11-ounce can mandarin oranges in juice, drained**
- ⅓ **cup chopped tomato**
- ⅓ **cup chopped avocado**
- 1 **tablespoon fresh lime juice**

- 2 **tuna steaks (about 8 ounces each), rinsed and patted dry**

Lightly spray a medium saucepan with cooking spray. Cook the onion and garlic over medium-high heat for 3 minutes, or until the onion is soft, stirring frequently.

Stir in the vinegar, brown sugar, and red pepper flakes. Cook for 2 to 3 minutes, or until the brown sugar is dissolved, stirring frequently. Remove from the heat.

Stir in the remaining pico de gallo ingredients. Set aside.

Meanwhile, lightly spray a large skillet with cooking spray. Heat over medium-high heat. Cook the fish for 5 minutes on each side, or to the desired doneness. Cut each piece in half. Serve with the pico de gallo.

tuna-noodle casserole

SERVES 5
1 cup per serving

PREPARATION TIME
10 minutes

COOKING TIME
40 minutes

PER SERVING
Calories 216
Total Fat 2.5 g
  Saturated Fat 0.5 g
  Trans Fat 0.0 g
  Polyunsaturated Fat 0.5 g
  Monounsaturated Fat 0.5 g
Cholesterol 28 mg
Sodium 400 mg
Carbohydrates 29 g
  Fiber 4 g
  Sugars 5 g
Protein 22 g
Dietary Exchanges
  1½ starch, 1 vegetable,
  2 very lean meat

You probably have a recipe for tuna-noodle casserole, but not like this one. It not only cuts down on the usual fat, sodium, and cholesterol and adds vegetables but also cuts out the step of boiling the noodles before baking the casserole. Less time and one less pot to wash!

1	10¾-ounce can low-fat condensed cream of chicken soup (lowest sodium available)
1	cup fat-free milk
2	5-ounce cans very low sodium white albacore tuna, packed in water, drained and flaked
10	ounces frozen mixed vegetables, such as peas, carrots, corn, and green beans, slightly thawed if needed to separate
3	ounces medium dried no-yolk noodles (about 2 cups), broken into small pieces
½	cup chopped onion
1	medium rib of celery, chopped
¼	cup snipped fresh parsley (optional)
¼	teaspoon paprika
⅛	teaspoon salt
⅛	teaspoon pepper

Preheat the oven to 375°F.

In a 2-quart glass casserole dish or 9-inch square glass baking dish, whisk together the soup and milk. Stir in the remaining ingredients.

Bake, covered, for 25 minutes. Stir. Bake, covered, for 15 minutes, or until the noodles are tender.

COOK'S TIP ON THAWING FOOD
To thaw frozen food that is not dense, put it in a colander and run it under cold water for a few seconds to several minutes, depending on whether you want the food partially or totally thawed. Put denser food, such as chicken breasts, in an airtight bag and soak for a few minutes in a large bowl of cold water.

tuna-topped barley
WITH KALAMATA-BASIL TOMATOES

SERVES 4
1 cup per serving

PREPARATION TIME
10 to 12 minutes

COOKING TIME
16 minutes

PER SERVING
Calories 255
Total Fat 9.0 g
  Saturated Fat 1.0 g
  Trans Fat 0.0 g
  Polyunsaturated Fat 1.5 g
  Monounsaturated Fat 5.5 g
Cholesterol 18 mg
Sodium 271 mg
Carbohydrates 32 g
  Fiber 5 g
  Sugars 2 g
Protein 16 g
Dietary Exchanges
  2 starch, 1½ very lean meat,
  1 fat

Barley combined with fresh spinach makes up the bottom layer of this one-dish Mediterranean dinner. That and the top layer—quickly cooked tomatoes, kalamata olives, and fresh basil—warm the tuna sandwiched in between.

1 cup uncooked quick-cooking barley
1½ ounces coarsely chopped spinach (about 1½ cups packed)
1 teaspoon bottled minced garlic or 2 medium garlic cloves, minced
1 tablespoon olive oil
1 cup grape tomatoes, quartered
15 kalamata olives, coarsely chopped
¼ cup chopped fresh basil (about ⅔ ounce) or 1 tablespoon dried, crumbled
1 6-ounce can very low sodium white albacore tuna, packed in water, drained and flaked

Prepare the barley using the package directions, omitting the salt. Drain well in a colander. Transfer the barley to a large shallow dish.

Add the spinach and garlic, tossing with tongs for 30 seconds, or until the spinach is slightly wilted. Cover to keep warm. Set aside.

In a medium nonstick skillet, heat the oil over medium-high heat, swirling to coat the bottom. Cook the tomatoes, olives, and basil for 2 minutes, or until the tomatoes are soft, stirring frequently. (Cooking this mixture just before layering all the ingredients helps keep the flavors "bright.")

Sprinkle the tuna over the barley mixture. Top with the tomato mixture. (The heat from the barley and tomato layers will slightly warm the tuna.)

dilled albacore cakes

SERVES 6
1 patty per serving

PREPARATION TIME
12 to 15 minutes

COOKING TIME
15 minutes

PER SERVING
Calories 126
Total Fat 5.0 g
  Saturated Fat 1.0 g
  Trans Fat 0.0 g
  Polyunsaturated Fat 2.5 g
  Monounsaturated Fat 1.0 g
Cholesterol 27 mg
Sodium 279 mg
Carbohydrates 5 g
  Fiber 1 g
  Sugars 1 g
Protein 16 g
Dietary Exchanges
  ½ starch, 2 lean meat

Fresh dillweed and Parmesan cheese amp up the flavor in this simple substitute for salmon patties.

Cooking spray
2   5-ounce cans very low sodium white albacore tuna, packed in water, drained and flaked
½   cup egg substitute
¼   cup plain dry bread crumbs (lowest sodium available)
¼   cup shredded or grated Parmesan cheese
2   medium green onions, sliced
1   tablespoon snipped fresh dillweed or ½ teaspoon dried, crumbled
½   teaspoon pepper (coarsely ground preferred)
⅓   cup light mayonnaise
½   teaspoon grated lemon zest
    Sprigs of fresh dillweed (optional)

Preheat the oven to 400°F. Lightly spray a medium shallow baking pan with cooking spray. Set aside.

In a medium bowl, stir together the tuna, egg substitute, bread crumbs, Parmesan, green onions, 1 tablespoon dillweed, and pepper. Shape into 6 patties. Arrange in a single layer in the baking pan.

Bake on one side for 15 minutes, or until lightly browned. Transfer to plates.

Meanwhile, in a small bowl, stir together the mayonnaise and lemon zest.

Spoon a dollop of the mayonnaise mixture onto each cake. Garnish with the sprigs of dillweed.

mussels

IN CREAMY WINE SAUCE

Serve these tender shellfish with chunks of whole-grain bread so you can soak up the creamy sauce.

  4 medium green onions, sliced
½ cup dry white wine (regular or nonalcoholic)
¼ teaspoon pepper
24 fresh debearded and rinsed medium mussels
½ cup fat-free evaporated milk
  2 tablespoons Dijon mustard (lowest sodium available)
1½ teaspoons all-purpose flour

In a Dutch oven, bring the green onions, wine, and pepper to a boil over high heat. Add the mussels. Cook, covered, for 3 to 5 minutes, or until the mussels have opened. Turn off the heat. Leaving the cooking liquid in the pot, transfer the mussels to a serving dish, discarding any mussels that did not open during cooking.

    In a small bowl, whisk together the milk, mustard, and flour. Whisk into the cooking liquid. Cook, still over high heat, for 5 minutes, or until the mixture is thickened to the desired consistency, whisking constantly. Pour over the mussels, stirring gently to coat.

COOK'S TIP ON MUSSELS

If the mussels you buy have not been cleaned and de-bearded, you can easily debeard them at home. Using your fingers, grasp the mossy-looking beard and pull it firmly until it comes away from the shell. Before cooking the mussels, tap each one to be sure the shell closes up tightly. If it doesn't, discard the mussel.

lemon-garlic scallops

SERVES 4
3 ounces scallops
per serving

PREPARATION TIME
10 minutes

MARINATING TIME
10 minutes

COOKING TIME
5 to 7 minutes

PER SERVING
Calories 132
Total Fat 3.0 g
  Saturated Fat 0.5 g
  Trans Fat 0.0 g
  Polyunsaturated Fat 0.5 g
  Monounsaturated Fat 1.5 g
Cholesterol 37 mg
Sodium 186 mg
Carbohydrates 6 g
  Fiber 1 g
  Sugars 1 g
Protein 19 g
Dietary Exchanges
  ½ other carbohydrate,
  3 very lean meat

At first glance, you may think there is too much garlic in this recipe, but the amount is perfectly balanced with the sweetness of the scallops and the tanginess of the lemon juice.

2   tablespoons fresh lemon juice
1   tablespoon bottled minced garlic or 6 medium garlic cloves, minced
2   teaspoons olive oil
⅛   teaspoon pepper
1   pound sea scallops, rinsed and patted dry
½   medium red bell pepper, cut into 2 × ⅛-inch strips
¼   cup sliced green onions

In a large shallow dish, whisk together the lemon juice, garlic, oil, and pepper. Add the scallops, turning to coat. Cover and refrigerate for 10 minutes, turning the scallops once halfway through.

Preheat a large nonstick skillet over medium-high heat. Cook the scallops with the marinade, bell pepper, and green onions for 4 to 6 minutes, or until the scallops are white on the outside and opaque almost to the center, and the sauce is bubbly. Turn the scallops once halfway through and stir the bell pepper and green onions occasionally. Don't overcook or the scallops will be dry and rubbery.

sherried seafood sauté

SERVES 4
½ cup per serving

PREPARATION TIME
10 minutes

COOKING TIME
6 to 7 minutes

PER SERVING

Calories 119
Total Fat 2.0 g
    Saturated Fat 0.0 g
    Trans Fat 0.0 g
    Polyunsaturated Fat 0.5 g
    Monounsaturated Fat 1.0 g
Cholesterol 116 mg
Sodium 294 mg
Carbohydrates 4 g
    Fiber 1 g
    Sugars 1 g
Protein 19 g
Dietary Exchanges
    2½ very lean meat

Easy but elegant, this entrée features fresh shrimp and lump crabmeat, which is cooked nuggets of white meat from the body of the crab. Serve this dish over spinach fettuccine or brown rice, with a dark green leafy salad.

Cooking spray
1   tablespoon light tub margarine
8   ounces peeled raw medium shrimp, rinsed and patted dry
½   cup preshredded carrot
3   medium green onions, sliced
1   teaspoon bottled minced garlic or 2 medium garlic cloves, minced
6   ounces lump crabmeat, flaked
2   tablespoons dry sherry or dry white wine (regular or nonalcoholic)

Lightly spray a large skillet with cooking spray. Melt the margarine over medium-high heat, swirling to coat the bottom. Cook the shrimp, carrot, green onions, and garlic for 3 minutes, or until the shrimp are pink on the outside, stirring frequently.

Stir in the crabmeat and sherry. Cook for 2 to 3 minutes, or until heated through, stirring constantly.

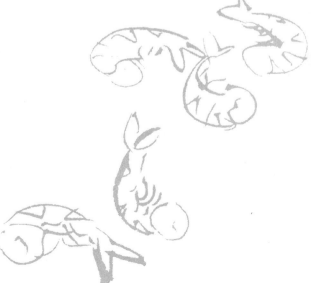

speedy shrimp and pasta

SERVES 4
1½ cups per serving

PREPARATION TIME
5 minutes

COOKING TIME
6 to 8 minutes

PER SERVING
Calories 352
Total Fat 4.5 g
  Saturated Fat 2.0 g
  Trans Fat 0.0 g
  Polyunsaturated Fat 0.5 g
  Monounsaturated Fat 0.5 g
Cholesterol 209 mg
Sodium 317 mg
Carbohydrates 48 g
  Fiber 5 g
  Sugars 5 g
Protein 30 g
Dietary Exchanges
  2½ starch, 2 vegetable,
  3 very lean meat

If you like the pasta and Parmesan cheese of fettuccine Alfredo and the veggies of pasta primavera, you'll love this little-bit-of-both combo! Using just one pot, you'll create a rich-tasting meal that provides protein, vegetables, and grain.

  1 **pound frozen peeled raw medium shrimp**
 14 **to 16 ounces frozen vegetables, any combination (stir-fry mixture preferred)**
  9 **ounces uncooked fresh fettuccine (lowest sodium available), halved crosswise and strands separated**
  ½ **cup water (plus more as needed)**
  ¼ **cup shredded or grated Parmesan or Romano cheese**
  ¼ **cup snipped fresh basil (about ⅔ ounce) or parsley Crushed red pepper flakes to taste (optional)**

In a large skillet, stir together the shrimp, vegetables, pasta, and water. Bring to a boil over high heat, stirring occasionally. Reduce the heat to medium and cook, covered, for 3 minutes, stirring occasionally and adding more water if needed to keep the pasta from sticking to the bottom of the pan. Cook, still covered, for 1 to 3 minutes, or until the shrimp are pink on the outside, the vegetables are tender-crisp, and the pasta is tender.

Serve sprinkled with the Parmesan, basil, and red pepper flakes.

COOK'S TIP ON FRESH PASTA
Check the refrigerated section of your grocery store when you're looking for fresh pasta. It is probably displayed with the refrigerated pasta sauces.

poultry

marinated hoisin chicken

PREPARATION TIME
6 minutes

MARINATING TIME
1 to 24 hours

COOKING TIME
45 to 55 minutes

PER SERVING
Calories 154
Total Fat 4.5 g
  Saturated Fat 1.0 g
  Trans Fat 0.0 g
  Polyunsaturated Fat 1.0 g
  Monounsaturated Fat 1.5 g
Cholesterol 73 mg
Sodium 173 mg
Carbohydrates 3 g
  Fiber 0 g
  Sugars 2 g
Protein 25 g
Dietary Exchanges
  3 lean meat

This so-easy chicken dish, with its dash of crunch from sesame seeds, is great paired with the very un-Italian Pasta and Sugar Snap Pea Salad (page 60).

  ¼ **cup hoisin sauce**
  ¼ **cup plain rice vinegar or cider vinegar**
  2 **tablespoons sesame seeds, dry-roasted**
  1¼ **pounds skinless chicken breast halves with bone, all visible fat discarded**

In a medium shallow glass dish, stir together the hoisin sauce, vinegar, and sesame seeds. Add the chicken, turning to coat. Cover and refrigerate for 1 to 24 hours, turning occasionally.

About an hour before serving time, preheat the oven to 375°F.

Arrange the chicken in a single layer in an 8-inch square glass baking dish, discarding the marinade.

Bake for 45 to 55 minutes, or until the chicken is no longer pink in the center.

COOK'S TIP ON HOISIN SAUCE
Hoisin sauce, sometimes referred to as Chinese ketchup, is a tongue-tingling mixture of fermented soybeans and seasonings. Look for jars of hoisin sauce in the Asian section of your grocery store. Although it has no true substitute, in a pinch you could replace the 2 tablespoons called for here with 1 tablespoon of dark molasses and 1 tablespoon of no-salt-added ketchup.

baked chicken
WITH WINTER VEGETABLES

SERVES 4

3 ounces chicken and
½ cup vegetables
per serving

PREPARATION TIME
15 minutes

COOKING TIME
1 hour 15 minutes to
1 hour 30 minutes

PER SERVING

Calories 313
Total Fat 3.5 g
  Saturated Fat 0.5 g
  Trans Fat 0.0 g
  Polyunsaturated Fat 0.5 g
  Monounsaturated Fat 1.0 g
Cholesterol 73 mg
Sodium 556 mg
Carbohydrates 43 g
  Fiber 6 g
  Sugars 9 g
Protein 29 g
Dietary Exchanges
  2½ starch, 2 vegetable,
  3 very lean meat

Warm up your family on a cold evening with this filling one-dish meal of chicken, seasonal vegetables, and gravy.

2 **skinless chicken breast halves with bone
   (7 to 8 ounces each), all visible fat discarded**
8 **small red potatoes, halved**
4 **large carrots, cut into 1-inch pieces**
1 **small acorn squash, quartered, seeds and strings
   discarded**
1 **medium onion or fennel bulb, cut into 8 wedges**
¼ **cup water**
¼ **teaspoon dried thyme, crumbled**
⅛ **teaspoon salt**
¼ **teaspoon pepper**
1 **cup bottled chicken gravy (lowest sodium
   available)**

Preheat the oven to 375°F.

Put the chicken in a 13 × 9 × 2-inch glass baking
dish or 3-quart glass casserole dish. Place the potatoes,
carrots, squash, and onion around the chicken. Pour the
water over all. Sprinkle with the thyme, salt, and pepper.

Bake, covered, for 1 hour 15 minutes to 1 hour
30 minutes, or until the chicken is no longer pink in
the center and the vegetables are tender. Transfer the
chicken to a cutting board. Cut each breast in half,
discarding the bones.

Shortly before serving time, using the directions on
the bottle, heat the gravy. Spoon over the cooked
chicken and vegetables.

COOK'S TIP ON FENNEL
*Fennel has a creamy white bulbous base, short pale green
stems, and feathery darker green leaves. Cooking fennel
makes its licorice-like flavor more delicate and its celery-
like texture softer.*

chicken-and-clementine kebabs
WITH PEACH GLAZE

SERVES 4
2 kebabs per serving

PREPARATION TIME
15 minutes

COOKING TIME
10 minutes

PER SERVING

Calories 214
Total Fat 3.0 g
  Saturated Fat 0.5 g
  Trans Fat 0.0 g
  Polyunsaturated Fat 0.5 g
  Monounsaturated Fat 1.0 g
Cholesterol 73 mg
Sodium 280 mg
Carbohydrates 21 g
  Fiber 2 g
  Sugars 14 g
Protein 25 g
Dietary Exchanges
  1 fruit, 1 vegetable,
  3 very lean meat

These colorful kebabs are pretty enough to serve at your next party. Part of the mandarin orange family, the clementines soften when they broil. That means you can enjoy the entire fruit, including the peel.

Cooking spray
1 pound boneless, skinless chicken breasts, all visible fat discarded, cut into 16 cubes
2 clementines, unpeeled, each cut into 8 wedges, seeds, if any, discarded
1 large red onion, cut into 16 wedges
1 medium yellow bell pepper, cut into 16 squares
¼ teaspoon salt
¼ teaspoon pepper
¼ cup all-fruit peach spread
2 tablespoons fresh orange juice

Soak eight 10-inch wooden skewers in cold water for at least 10 minutes to keep them from charring, or use metal skewers.

Meanwhile, preheat the broiler. Lightly spray a broiler pan and rack with cooking spray. Set aside.

For each kebab, skewer in any order two each of the chicken cubes, clementine wedges, onion wedges, and bell pepper squares. Sprinkle the kebabs on all sides with the salt and pepper.

Broil the kebabs at least 4 inches from the heat for 8 minutes, turning once halfway through. Remove the broiler pan from the oven.

Meanwhile, in a small bowl, whisk together the all-fruit spread and orange juice. Spoon 2 tablespoons of the mixture into a small dish and reserve for drizzling.

Brush the kebabs with the all-fruit spread mixture from the small bowl. Broil for 2 minutes, or until the chicken is no longer pink in the center. Drizzle with the reserved 2 tablespoons all-fruit spread mixture.

baked chicken
WITH CRUNCHY BASIL-PARMESAN PESTO

SERVES 6
3 ounces chicken and
1½ teaspoons pesto
per serving
(plus heaping
½ cup pesto remaining)

PREPARATION TIME
18 to 20 minutes

COOKING TIME
20 to 30 minutes

PER SERVING

Calories 167
Total Fat 5.0 g
 Saturated Fat 1.0 g
 Trans Fat 0.0 g
 Polyunsaturated Fat 1.0 g
 Monounsaturated Fat 2.0 g
Cholesterol 74 mg
Sodium 188 mg
Carbohydrates 4 g
 Fiber 0 g
 Sugars 0 g
Protein 25 g
Dietary Exchanges
 3 lean meat

*The aromatic pesto keeps the chicken moist during baking
and helps hold the cornflake crumbs in place. You'll have
enough pesto left over to make Layered Pesto Spread
(page 34) or Pesto Pork Pinwheels (page 162), or to toss
with piping-hot whole-grain pasta.*

PESTO
  1 cup firmly packed fresh basil (about 3 ounces)
  ½ cup firmly packed fresh Italian (flat-leaf) parsley
  ½ cup shredded or grated Parmesan cheese
  ¼ cup walnuts
  1 teaspoon bottled minced garlic or 2 medium
     garlic cloves, minced
  2 tablespoons olive oil (extra-virgin preferred)
  2 tablespoons fat-free, low-sodium chicken broth

CHICKEN
1½ pounds boneless, skinless chicken breast halves,
     all visible fat discarded
  ¼ cup cornflake crumbs

  1 large lemon or 2 medium limes, each cut into
     6 wedges (optional)

Preheat the oven to 375°F.

In a food processor or blender, process the basil,
parsley, Parmesan, walnuts, and garlic to a paste,
scraping the side as needed.

With the processor running, gradually add the oil
and broth. Process until smooth. Transfer 3 tablespoons
of the pesto to a small bowl. Transfer the remaining
pesto to a small airtight container and refrigerate for
another use.

Put the chicken in a shallow baking pan large enough
to hold it in a single layer. Lightly brush the top with
3 tablespoons pesto. Sprinkle with the cornflake
crumbs.

Bake for 20 to 30 minutes, or until the chicken is no
longer pink in the center. Serve with the lemon wedges
for squeezing over the chicken.

chinese-style chicken

SERVES 4
3 ounces chicken and
1 tablespoon sauce
per serving

PREPARATION TIME
8 minutes

COOKING TIME
30 to 35 minutes

OR

MICROWAVE TIME
11 to 14 minutes

PER SERVING
Calories 158
Total Fat 4.0 g
  Saturated Fat 1.0 g
  Trans Fat 0.0 g
  Polyunsaturated Fat 1.0 g
  Monounsaturated Fat 1.5 g
Cholesterol 73 mg
Sodium 327 mg
Carbohydrates 4 g
  Fiber 0 g
  Sugars 2 g
Protein 25 g
Dietary Exchanges
  3 lean meat

Instead of buying Chinese takeout, why not stay in and enjoy this Asian-inspired dish? You can prep and cook it in about the same time it would take to call in your order and drive to pick it up or have it delivered.

4   boneless, skinless chicken breast halves (about 4 ounces each), all visible fat discarded
2   tablespoons soy sauce (lowest sodium available)
2   tablespoons plain rice vinegar or cider vinegar
2   tablespoons dry sherry or fresh orange juice
1   teaspoon toasted sesame oil
1   teaspoon honey
½   teaspoon bottled minced garlic or 1 medium garlic clove, minced
1   teaspoon cornstarch
1   tablespoon fresh orange juice or water

Preheat the oven to 350°F.

Arrange the chicken in a single layer in an 8-inch square baking dish.

In a small bowl, stir together the soy sauce, vinegar, sherry, sesame oil, honey, and garlic. Pour over the chicken.

Bake for 25 to 30 minutes, or until the chicken is no longer pink in the center. Transfer the chicken to a large plate. Cover to keep warm. Pour the sauce into a small saucepan.

Put the cornstarch in a small bowl. Add the orange juice, whisking to dissolve. Pour into the sauce. Cook over medium heat for 5 minutes, or until thickened and bubbly, whisking constantly. Spoon over the chicken.

MICROWAVE METHOD

Arrange the chicken in a microwaveable dish large enough to hold it in a single layer. Combine the soy sauce mixture as directed. Pour over the chicken. Microwave, covered and vented, on 100 percent power (high) for 8 to 10 minutes, or until the chicken is no longer pink in the center. Transfer the chicken to a large plate. Cover to keep warm.

Pour the sauce into a 2-cup glass measuring cup. Put the cornstarch in a small bowl. Add the orange juice, whisking to dissolve. Pour into the sauce. Microwave on 100 percent power (high) for 1 to 2 minutes, or until thickened and bubbly, stirring every 30 seconds. Spoon over the chicken.

COOK'S TIP

When a recipe calls for sherry or wine, don't use cooking sherry or cooking wine; they are very salty. If you don't want to use the real thing, substitute nonalcoholic wine, fruit juice, or water.

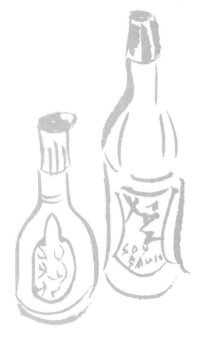

grilled chicken
WITH STRAWBERRY-FIG SAUCE

SERVES 4
3 ounces chicken and
¼ cup sauce per serving

PREPARATION TIME
20 minutes

COOKING TIME
12 to 15 minutes

PER SERVING
Calories 223
Total Fat 3.5 g
  Saturated Fat 0.5 g
  Trans Fat 0.0 g
  Polyunsaturated Fat 0.5 g
  Monounsaturated Fat 1.0 g
Cholesterol 73 mg
Sodium 145 mg
Carbohydrates 23 g
  Fiber 4 g
  Sugars 16 g
Protein 26 g
Dietary Exchanges
  1½ fruit, 3 lean meat

Zesty spices that are common in Moroccan cuisine accent this colorful dish. A sweet-tangy fruit sauce provides the perfect balance.

Cooking spray
1 teaspoon paprika
1 teaspoon ground cumin
½ teaspoon ground ginger
¼ teaspoon pepper
1 tablespoon fresh lemon juice
1 pound boneless, skinless chicken breast halves, all visible fat discarded
½ cup chopped dried figs
½ cup fat-free, low-sodium chicken broth
1 medium shallot, sliced
¼ cup fresh orange juice
⅛ teaspoon ground cinnamon
1 pint strawberries, hulled and coarsely chopped (about 2 cups)
1 tablespoon balsamic vinegar
1 tablespoon snipped fresh parsley

Preheat the grill on medium. Lightly spray the grill rack with cooking spray.

In a small bowl, stir together the paprika, cumin, ginger, and pepper. Set aside.

Put the lemon juice in a medium dish. Add the chicken, turning to coat. Sprinkle the paprika mixture over both sides of the chicken. Using your fingertips, gently press the mixture so it adheres to the chicken.

Grill the chicken for 12 to 15 minutes, or until no longer pink in the center, turning once halfway through.

Meanwhile, in a medium skillet, stir together the figs, broth, shallot, orange juice, and cinnamon. Bring to a boil over medium-high heat. Boil for 6 minutes, or until most of the liquid is evaporated, stirring occasionally. Remove from the heat.

Stir in the strawberries and vinegar. Let stand for 3 to 5 minutes, or until slightly cooled. Serve the sauce over the chicken. Sprinkle with the parsley.

skillet chicken

WITH DRIED BERRIES

SERVES 4

3 ounces chicken and ¼ cup sauce per serving

PREPARATION TIME

5 minutes

COOKING TIME

16 to 17 minutes

PER SERVING

WITH WINE

Calories 184
Total Fat 3.0 g
  Saturated Fat 0.5 g
  Trans Fat 0.0 g
  Polyunsaturated Fat 0.5 g
  Monounsaturated Fat 1.0 g
Cholesterol 73 mg
Sodium 135 mg
Carbohydrates 8 g
  Fiber 1 g
  Sugars 6 g
Protein 24 g
Dietary Exchanges
  ½ fruit, 3 very lean meat

WITH CRANBERRY
JUICE COCKTAIL

Calories 164
Total Fat 3.0 g
  Saturated Fat 0.5 g
  Trans Fat 0.0 g
  Polyunsaturated Fat 0.5 g
  Monounsaturated Fat 1.0 g
Cholesterol 73 mg
Sodium 144 mg
Carbohydrates 9 g
  Fiber 1 g
  Sugars 8 g
Protein 24 g
Dietary Exchanges
  ½ fruit, 3 very lean meat

Decisions, decisions! Would you rather have the richer, more robust sauce that you get with red wine, or do you prefer the slightly sweet and fruity sauce that you get with cranberry juice cocktail? Choosing your liquid, then your favorite dried fruit, is the hard part—the actual cooking is a snap.

Cooking spray

4   boneless, skinless chicken breast halves (about 4 ounces each), all visible fat discarded

⅔ cup dry red wine (regular or nonalcoholic) or light cranberry juice cocktail

¼ cup sweetened dried cranberries, dried blueberries, dried cherries, or mixed dried fruit bits

½ teaspoon dried thyme, crumbled

1   teaspoon cornstarch

1   tablespoon water

Lightly spray a large skillet with cooking spray. Heat over medium-high heat. Cook the chicken for 1 minute on each side (the chicken won't be done at this point). Transfer to a large plate. Set aside.

In the same skillet, stir together the wine, cranberries, and thyme. Increase the heat to high and bring to a boil.

Add the chicken, turning to coat. Reduce the heat and simmer, covered, for about 5 minutes, or until the chicken is no longer pink in the center. Transfer to a platter, leaving the sauce in the skillet. Cover to keep warm.

Put the cornstarch in a small bowl. Add the water, whisking to dissolve. Whisk into the sauce. Cook over medium heat for 5 minutes, or until thickened and bubbly, whisking constantly. Spoon over the chicken.

chicken

WITH FRESH FRUIT AND VEGGIE SALSA

SERVES 4
3 ounces chicken and
¼ cup salsa per serving

PREPARATION TIME
10 minutes

COOKING TIME
10 minutes

PER SERVING
Calories 150
Total Fat 3.0 g
    Saturated Fat 0.5 g
    Trans Fat 0.0 g
    Polyunsaturated Fat 0.5 g
    Monounsaturated Fat 1.0 g
Cholesterol 73 mg
Sodium 279 mg
Carbohydrates 5 g
    Fiber 1 g
    Sugars 3 g
Protein 25 g
Dietary Exchanges
    ½ fruit, 3 very lean meat

Perfect for a summer lunch or dinner on the patio, this entrée features an unusual salsa that bursts with the fresh flavors of fruit, tomato, and red onion.

Cooking spray

SALSA
½   cup chopped fresh apricots, peaches, or nectarines
1   small tomato, chopped
¼   cup chopped red onion
2   tablespoons fresh lemon juice
¼   teaspoon salt
¼   teaspoon finely grated peeled gingerroot
¼   teaspoon bottled minced garlic or ½ medium garlic clove, minced

4   boneless, skinless chicken breast halves (about 4 ounces each), all visible fat discarded

Preheat the grill on medium high or preheat the broiler. Lightly spray the grill rack or the broiler pan and rack with cooking spray.

In a medium bowl, stir together the salsa ingredients. Set aside.

Grill the chicken or broil 4 to 5 inches from the heat for 5 minutes, or until lightly browned. Turn over. Grill or broil for 5 minutes, or until no longer pink in the center. Serve with the salsa.

COOK'S TIP
You can make the salsa up to 24 hours in advance. Transfer it to an airtight container and refrigerate. For the best flavor, bring the salsa to room temperature before serving.

lemony chicken

WITH TARRAGON OIL

SERVES 4
3 ounces chicken and
1 tablespoon tarragon oil
per serving

PREPARATION TIME
6 to 7 minutes

COOKING TIME
6 to 8 minutes

PER SERVING
Calories 192
Total Fat 9.5 g
 Saturated Fat 1.5 g
 Trans Fat 0.0 g
 Polyunsaturated Fat 1.0 g
 Monounsaturated Fat 6.0 g
Cholesterol 73 mg
Sodium 277 mg
Carbohydrates 1 g
 Fiber 0 g
 Sugars 0 g
Protein 24 g
Dietary Exchanges
 3 lean meat

Although you use only a small amount of it, tarragon, an assertive herb with a sweet, aniselike flavor, is the star of the show in this dish. A complementary side dish is Citrus Kale with Dried Cranberries (page 215).

  Cooking spray
2 tablespoons olive oil (extra-virgin preferred)
2 tablespoons fresh lemon juice
½ teaspoon dried tarragon, crumbled
¼ teaspoon pepper (coarsely ground preferred)
¼ teaspoon salt
4 boneless, skinless chicken breast halves (about 4 ounces each), all visible fat discarded, flattened to ½-inch thickness
1½ teaspoons salt-free grilling seasoning blend

If grilling, lightly spray a grill rack with cooking spray. Preheat the grill on medium high. If cooking on the stove, lightly spray a large skillet. Set aside.

In a small bowl, whisk together the oil, lemon juice, tarragon, pepper, and salt. Set aside.

Sprinkle the chicken on both sides with the seasoning blend. Using your fingertips, gently press the seasonings so they adhere to the chicken.

If grilling, grill the chicken for 4 minutes. Turn over and grill for 2 to 4 minutes, or until no longer pink in the center. If using the stovetop, cook the chicken over medium-high heat for 4 minutes. Turn over and cook for 2 minutes, or until no longer pink in the center. Transfer the chicken to a platter.

Just before serving, whisk the oil mixture. Spoon over the chicken.

cheesy oven-fried chicken

SERVES 4
3 ounces chicken
per serving

PREPARATION TIME
10 minutes

COOKING TIME
7 to 9 minutes

PER SERVING
Calories 224
Total Fat 5.5 g
  Saturated Fat 2.5 g
  Trans Fat 0.0 g
  Polyunsaturated Fat 0.5 g
  Monounsaturated Fat 1.5 g
Cholesterol 80 mg
Sodium 327 mg
Carbohydrates 11 g
  Fiber 1 g
  Sugars 1 g
Protein 30 g
Dietary Exchanges
  1 starch, 3 lean meat

These chicken nuggets are just right for little hands and big appetites. Serve the nuggets with Homemade Corn Tortilla Chips (page 40) and a salad or fresh fruit.

Cooking spray
2   tablespoons fat-free milk
1   cup plain panko (Japanese bread crumbs)
½   cup shredded or grated Parmesan cheese
½ to ¾ teaspoon dried basil, crumbled
⅛   teaspoon pepper
1   pound boneless, skinless chicken tenders, all visible fat discarded, cut into bite-size pieces

Preheat the oven to 400°F. Lightly spray a shallow baking pan with cooking spray.

Put the milk in a small shallow dish.

In a medium shallow dish, stir together the panko, Parmesan, basil, and pepper.

Put the dishes and baking pan in a row, assembly-line fashion. Dip several pieces of chicken in the milk, turning to coat and letting any excess drip off. Dip in the panko mixture, turning to coat and gently shaking off any excess. Transfer to the pan. Repeat with the remaining chicken, arranging the pieces in a single layer.

Bake for 7 to 9 minutes, or until the chicken is no longer pink in the center and the crust begins to brown.

chicken
WITH LEEKS AND TOMATOES

SERVES 4
3 ounces chicken and
^{2}/$_3$ cup vegetables
per serving

PREPARATION TIME
12 minutes

COOKING TIME
18 to 22 minutes

PER SERVING
Calories 177
Total Fat 5.5 g
  Saturated Fat 1.0 g
  Trans Fat 0.0 g
  Polyunsaturated Fat 1.0 g
  Monounsaturated Fat 2.5 g
Cholesterol 73 mg
Sodium 218 mg
Carbohydrates 6 g
  Fiber 1 g
  Sugars 3 g
Protein 25 g
Dietary Exchanges
  1 vegetable, 3 lean meat

Fresh vegetables, sage, and lemon combine to add lots of visual appeal and flavor to this dish. Try it with Toasted Barley Pilaf (page 208).

1   **pound boneless, skinless chicken breast halves, all visible fat discarded, flattened to ¼-inch thickness**
¼   **teaspoon pepper**
⅛   **teaspoon salt**
2   **teaspoons olive oil**
1   **medium leek**
1   **cup halved red or yellow cherry tomatoes, or a combination**
¼   **cup fat-free, low-sodium chicken broth**
1   **tablespoon snipped fresh sage or 1 teaspoon dried sage**
1   **medium lemon, cut into 4 wedges**

Sprinkle both sides of the chicken with the pepper and salt. Using your fingertips, gently press the seasonings so they adhere to the chicken.

In a large nonstick skillet, heat the oil over medium-high heat, swirling to coat the bottom. Put the chicken in the skillet. Reduce the heat to medium. Cook for 8 to 10 minutes, or until the chicken is no longer pink in the center, turning once halfway through. Transfer to a large plate. Cover to keep warm.

Meanwhile, trim the leek, discarding all the green part except a small amount of the light green. Slice the light green part. Halve and slice the white part. (You should have about 1¼ cups total.) Set aside.

After transferring the chicken to the plate, cook the leek in the same skillet over medium-high heat for 3 minutes, stirring occasionally.

Stir in the tomatoes. Cook for 2 minutes, stirring occasionally.

Stir in the broth and bring to a boil. Boil for 3 to 4 minutes, or until most of the liquid is evaporated.

Stir in the sage. Spoon the sauce onto plates. Top with the chicken. Serve with the lemon wedges to squeeze over the chicken.

lemon-pepper chicken
OVER PASTA

SERVES 4
3 ounces chicken and
½ cup pasta per serving

PREPARATION TIME
15 minutes

COOKING TIME
15 to 20 minutes

OR

MICROWAVE TIME
8 to 10 minutes

PER SERVING
Calories 259
Total Fat 4.5 g
  Saturated Fat 1.0 g
  Trans Fat 0.0 g
  Polyunsaturated Fat 1.0 g
  Monounsaturated Fat 1.5 g
Cholesterol 73 mg
Sodium 341 mg
Carbohydrates 25 g
  Fiber 2 g
  Sugars 4 g
Protein 29 g
Dietary Exchanges
  1½ starch, 3 very lean meat

Adding a small amount of a fresh herb really perks up bottled marinara sauce. In this recipe, the bright red sauce provides a nice contrast to the peppered chicken and the green pasta.

4 boneless, skinless chicken breast halves (about 4 ounces each), all visible fat discarded
½ medium lemon
   Pepper to taste
4 ounces dried spinach linguine or fettuccine
1 cup marinara sauce (lowest sodium available), at room temperature
2 tablespoons snipped fresh basil or parsley

Preheat the oven to 375°F.

Arrange the chicken in a glass baking dish large enough to hold it in a single layer. Squeeze the lemon half over the chicken. Sprinkle generously with the pepper. Using your fingertips, gently press the pepper so it adheres to the chicken.

Bake, covered, for 15 to 20 minutes, or until the chicken is no longer pink in the center. Cut the chicken into thick strips.

Meanwhile, prepare the pasta using the package directions, omitting the salt. Drain well in a colander. Return the pan to the burner (turn off the heat), and return the pasta to the pan. Add the marinara sauce and basil, stirring to coat. Cover to keep warm.

When the chicken is ready, spoon the pasta mixture onto plates. Top with the chicken.

MICROWAVE METHOD

Prepare the recipe as directed, but microwave the chicken, covered and vented, on 100 percent power (high) for 8 to 10 minutes, or until no longer pink in the center.

coriander-coated chicken

SERVES 4
3 ounces chicken
per serving

PREPARATION TIME
5 minutes

COOKING TIME
13 to 14 minutes

PER SERVING
Calories 172
Total Fat 3.5 g
  Saturated Fat 0.5 g
  Trans Fat 0.0 g
  Polyunsaturated Fat 0.5 g
  Monounsaturated Fat 1.0 g
Cholesterol 73 mg
Sodium 279 mg
Carbohydrates 10 g
  Fiber 1 g
  Sugars 9 g
Protein 25 g
Dietary Exchanges
  ½ other carbohydrate,
  3 very lean meat

A coating of honey holds aromatic seasonings and crunchy sesame seeds in place as these chicken breasts quickly bake.

  Cooking spray
4 **boneless, skinless chicken breast halves (about 4 ounces each), all visible fat discarded**
2 **tablespoons honey**
2 **teaspoons ground coriander**
1 **to 2 teaspoons ground cumin**
1 **teaspoon sesame seeds, dry-roasted**
1 **teaspoon snipped fresh thyme or ¼ teaspoon dried, crumbled**
¼ **teaspoon salt**
¼ **to ½ teaspoon pepper (coarsely ground preferred)**

Preheat the oven to 350°F.

Lightly spray a large ovenproof skillet with cooking spray. (If you don't have an ovenproof skillet, cook the chicken in a regular skillet and transfer to a shallow baking pan.) Heat the skillet over medium-high heat. Cook the chicken for 1 minute on each side, or until browned (the chicken won't be done at this point). Remove from the heat, leaving the chicken in the skillet.

Lightly brush the honey over the chicken.

In a small bowl, stir together the remaining ingredients. Sprinkle over the chicken.

Bake for 10 minutes, or until the chicken is no longer pink in the center.

spicy peanut chicken

SERVES 4
¾ cup chicken mixture
and ½ cup rice
per serving

PREPARATION TIME
10 minutes

COOKING TIME
7 to 9 minutes

MICROWAVE TIME
2½ to 4 minutes

PER SERVING

Calories 303
Total Fat 10.0 g
  Saturated Fat 1.5 g
  Trans Fat 0.0 g
  Polyunsaturated Fat 2.5 g
  Monounsaturated Fat 4.0 g
Cholesterol 73 mg
Sodium 256 mg
Carbohydrates 23 g
  Fiber 3 g
  Sugars 2 g
Protein 30 g
Dietary Exchanges
  1½ starch, 3 lean meat

Make this Thai-inspired dish as spicy as you like by using your favorite mild, medium, or hot salsa.

Cooking spray

1 **pound boneless, skinless chicken breasts, all visible fat discarded, cut into bite-size pieces**

1 **medium green bell pepper, cut into bite-size pieces**

10 **ounces frozen brown rice**

½ **cup Chunky Salsa (page 32) or commercial salsa (lowest sodium available)**

1 **tablespoon peanut butter (lowest sodium available)**

1 **tablespoon soy sauce (lowest sodium available)**

1 **teaspoon bottled minced garlic or 2 medium garlic cloves, minced**

1 **teaspoon finely grated peeled gingerroot**

¼ **cup coarsely chopped peanuts, dry-roasted**

¼ **cup snipped fresh basil (about ⅔ ounce)**

Lightly spray a large skillet with cooking spray. Heat over medium-high heat. Cook the chicken and bell pepper for 3 to 5 minutes, or until the chicken is no longer pink in the center, stirring occasionally.

Using the package directions, microwave the rice. Set aside.

Meanwhile, stir the salsa, peanut butter, soy sauce, garlic, and gingerroot into the chicken mixture. Cook for 3 minutes, or until thickened and bubbly, stirring constantly.

Spoon the rice onto plates. Spoon the chicken mixture on top. Sprinkle with the peanuts and basil.

barbecue-simmered chicken chunks

SERVES 4

½ cup per serving

PREPARATION TIME

4 minutes

COOKING TIME

6 minutes

PER SERVING

Calories 199
Total Fat 3.0 g
  Saturated Fat 0.5 g
  Trans Fat 0.0 g
  Polyunsaturated Fat 0.5 g
  Monounsaturated Fat 1.0 g
Cholesterol 73 mg
Sodium 237 mg
Carbohydrates 17 g
  Fiber 0 g
  Sugars 14 g
Protein 24 g
Dietary Exchanges
  1 other carbohydrate,
  3 very lean meat

Stretching bottled barbecue sauce by adding all-fruit spread is a clever way to cut sodium and add flavor. Serve the tangy poultry mixture in this recipe with sides of Crisp Skin-On Oven Fries (page 222) and green beans.

Cooking spray
1 pound boneless, skinless chicken breasts, all visible fat discarded, cut into bite-size pieces
¼ cup barbecue sauce (lowest sodium available)
¼ cup all-fruit spread, such as red plum or apricot

Lightly spray a large skillet with cooking spray. Heat over medium-high heat. Cook the chicken for 3 minutes, stirring occasionally.

Stir in the barbecue sauce and all-fruit spread. Cook for 3 minutes, or until the chicken is no longer pink in the center and the sauce is heated through, stirring frequently.

baked dijon chicken

SERVES 4
3 ounces chicken
per serving

PREPARATION TIME
6 minutes

COOKING TIME
15 to 20 minutes

OR

MICROWAVE TIME
6 to 8 minutes

PER SERVING
Calories 136
Total Fat 3.0 g
  Saturated Fat 0.5 g
  Trans Fat 0.0 g
  Polyunsaturated Fat 0.5 g
  Monounsaturated Fat 1.0 g
Cholesterol 73 mg
Sodium 208 mg
Carbohydrates 1 g
  Fiber 0 g
  Sugars 0 g
Protein 24 g
Dietary Exchanges
  3 very lean meat

Haute cuisine gets fast-tracked with this superbly easy version of a French favorite.

Cooking spray
4 **boneless, skinless chicken breast halves (about 4 ounces each), all visible fat discarded**
1 **tablespoon Dijon or coarse-grain mustard (lowest sodium available)**
2 **teaspoons fresh lemon or lime juice**
½ **teaspoon bottled minced garlic or 1 medium garlic clove, minced**
⅛ **teaspoon pepper**

Preheat the oven to 375°F. Lightly spray a 9-inch square glass baking dish with cooking spray.

Arrange the chicken in a single layer in the dish.

In a small bowl, stir together the remaining ingredients. Spread over the top of the chicken.

Bake for 15 to 20 minutes, or until the chicken is no longer pink in the center.

MICROWAVE METHOD

Arrange the chicken in the glass baking dish so the thicker portions are toward the edges of the dish. Spread the mustard mixture over the chicken as directed. Microwave, covered, on 100 percent power (high) for 3 to 4 minutes on each side, or until the chicken is no longer pink in the center.

poultry and mango stir-fry

SERVES 4
¾ cup per serving

PREPARATION TIME
6 minutes

COOKING TIME
10 to 13 minutes

PER SERVING
Calories 203
Total Fat 6.5 g
  Saturated Fat 1.0 g
  Trans Fat 0.0 g
  Polyunsaturated Fat 1.0 g
  Monounsaturated Fat 2.5 g
Cholesterol 73 mg
Sodium 201 mg
Carbohydrates 10 g
  Fiber 1 g
  Sugars 8 g
Protein 26 g
Dietary Exchanges
  ½ fruit, 3 lean meat

This dish is so easy to make that you'll want to serve it again and again. To keep it from becoming boring, you can vary the flavor of the stir-fry sauce, use peaches instead of mango, or substitute walnuts for the almonds.

Cooking spray
1 **pound boneless, skinless chicken breasts, all visible fat discarded, cut into bite-size pieces**
2 **tablespoons Asian-style stir-fry sauce (lowest sodium available)**
1 **cup coarsely chopped mango, drained and patted dry if bottled**
¼ **cup sliced almonds, dry-roasted**

Lightly spray a large skillet with cooking spray. Heat over medium-high heat. Cook the chicken for 3 to 5 minutes, or until no longer pink in the center, stirring occasionally. Remove from the heat.

Stir in the stir-fry sauce. Gently stir in the mango. Cook over medium heat for 5 minutes, or until heated through, stirring frequently. Serve sprinkled with the almonds.

COOK'S TIP
You can save a lot of time by buying a jar of sliced mangoes in your grocer's produce department and using part of the fruit for this recipe. Use some of the remaining mangoes in Grilled Salmon with Mango-Lime Cream Sauce (page 79) and enjoy the rest for healthy snacking.

lemon-sauced chicken

WITH ASPARAGUS

SERVES 4
1 cup per serving

PREPARATION TIME
10 minutes

COOKING TIME
12 to 14 minutes

PER SERVING
Calories 191
Total Fat 5.5 g
  Saturated Fat 1.0 g
  Trans Fat 0.0 g
  Polyunsaturated Fat 1.0 g
  Monounsaturated Fat 2.5 g
Cholesterol 73 mg
Sodium 243 mg
Carbohydrates 8 g
  Fiber 2 g
  Sugars 2 g
Protein 27 g
Dietary Exchanges
  1 vegetable, 3 lean meat

Serve this piquant chicken-and-vegetable stir-fry with whole-grain pasta, then end your meal beautifully with the sweet-tart flavors of Balsamic Berries Brûlée (page 250).

SAUCE

½ cup fat-free, low-sodium chicken broth
1 teaspoon finely grated lemon zest
2 tablespoons fresh lemon juice
1 tablespoon cornstarch
1 tablespoon soy sauce (lowest sodium available)
1 teaspoon sugar
¼ teaspoon pepper

1 teaspoon canola or corn oil and 1 teaspoon canola or corn oil, divided use
10 ounces frozen cut asparagus or broccoli florets, thawed and patted dry
1 small red bell pepper, cut into bite-size pieces
1 pound boneless, skinless chicken breasts, all visible fat discarded, cut into bite-size pieces

In a small bowl, whisk together the sauce ingredients until the cornstarch is dissolved. Set aside.

In a large skillet, heat 1 teaspoon oil over high heat, swirling to coat the bottom. Cook the asparagus and bell pepper for 1 minute, stirring constantly. Transfer to a large plate. Set aside.

In the same skillet, heat the remaining 1 teaspoon oil over high heat, swirling to coat the bottom. Cook the chicken for 3 to 5 minutes, or until no longer pink in the center, stirring constantly. Make a well in the center.

Stir the sauce. Pour into the well in the skillet. Cook for 4 minutes, or until the sauce is thickened and bubbly, stirring constantly.

Return the asparagus mixture to the skillet, stirring to coat.

light chicken chili

SERVES 6
¾ cup per serving

PREPARATION TIME
8 minutes

COOKING TIME
15 to 18 minutes

PER SERVING

Calories 227
Total Fat 2.0 g
  Saturated Fat 0.5 g
  Trans Fat 0.0 g
  Polyunsaturated Fat 0.5 g
  Monounsaturated Fat 0.5 g
Cholesterol 48 mg
Sodium 281 mg
Carbohydrates 26 g
  Fiber 7 g
  Sugars 6 g
Protein 25 g
Dietary Exchanges
  1½ starch, 3 very lean meat

Celebrate the coming of fall and cooler weather with the comfort of this white chili. It uses both mashed and whole beans, one kind for thickening and the other for texture.

Cooking spray
1 **pound boneless, skinless chicken breasts, all visible fat discarded, cut into bite-size pieces**
1 **medium onion, chopped**
1 **teaspoon bottled minced garlic or 2 medium garlic cloves, minced**
2 **cups fat-free, low-sodium chicken broth**
1 **4-ounce can chopped green chiles, drained**
1 **teaspoon ground cumin**
½ **teaspoon pepper (white preferred)**
¼ **teaspoon salt**
2 **15.5-ounce cans no-salt-added navy or Great Northern beans, rinsed and drained, divided use**

Lightly spray a Dutch oven with cooking spray. Cook the chicken, onion, and garlic over medium-high heat for 3 to 5 minutes, or until the chicken is no longer pink in the center, stirring occasionally.

Stir in the remaining ingredients except the beans. Bring to a boil. Reduce the heat and simmer for 5 minutes.

Meanwhile, in a medium bowl, mash one can of the beans until smooth.

When the chili has simmered, stir in the mashed beans and the remaining can of whole beans. Simmer for 5 minutes, or until heated through.

chicken and rice

WITH HERBS

SERVES 4
3 ounces chicken and
¾ cup rice mixture
per serving

PREPARATION TIME
5 minutes

COOKING TIME
30 to 36 minutes

PER SERVING
Calories 320
Total Fat 5.5 g
  Saturated Fat 1.0 g
  Trans Fat 0.0 g
  Polyunsaturated Fat 1.0 g
  Monounsaturated Fat 2.5 g
Cholesterol 73 mg
Sodium 298 mg
Carbohydrates 33 g
  Fiber 2 g
  Sugars 4 g
Protein 29 g
Dietary Exchanges
  2 starch, 1 vegetable,
  3 very lean meat

This easy dish incorporates the flavors of roast chicken and mushroom-herb stuffing but takes only a fraction of the time.

2   teaspoons olive oil
4   boneless, skinless chicken breast halves (about
    4 ounces each), all visible fat discarded
1   large onion, chopped
1   teaspoon bottled minced garlic or 2 medium
    garlic cloves, minced
8   ounces presliced button mushrooms
1   cup fat-free, low-sodium chicken broth
½   cup dry white wine (regular or nonalcoholic)
¼   teaspoon salt
¼   teaspoon dried thyme, crumbled
⅛   teaspoon dried basil, crumbled
¾   cup uncooked white rice

In a large nonstick skillet, heat the oil over medium-high heat, swirling to coat the bottom. Cook the chicken for 2 minutes on each side, or until lightly browned (the chicken won't be done at this point). Transfer to a plate. Set aside.

In the same skillet, stir together the onion and garlic. Cook over medium heat for 2 minutes. Stir in the mushrooms. Cook for 3 to 4 minutes, or until the onion is soft, stirring occasionally.

Pour the broth and wine into the skillet, scraping to dislodge any browned bits. Stir in the salt, thyme, and basil. Increase the heat to medium high and bring to a simmer.

Stir in the rice. Top with the chicken. Return to a simmer. Reduce the heat and simmer, covered, for 15 to 20 minutes, or until the chicken is no longer pink in the center and the rice is tender.

plum good chicken

SERVES 4
3 ounces chicken and
1¼ cups vegetable
mixture per serving

PREPARATION TIME
15 minutes

COOKING TIME
50 minutes

PER SERVING
Calories 419
Total Fat 11.0 g
  Saturated Fat 4.5 g
  Trans Fat 0.0 g
  Polyunsaturated Fat 1.5 g
  Monounsaturated Fat 4.0 g
Cholesterol 73 mg
Sodium 559 mg
Carbohydrates 48 g
  Fiber 4 g
  Sugars 13 g
Protein 33 g
Dietary Exchanges
  1½ starch, 2 vegetable,
  1 other carbohydrate,
  3 lean meat, 1 fat

This Asian-inspired one-dish meal boasts a medley of noodles, vegetables, and chicken topped with a tasty plum sauce. There's no need to prepare the noodles separately—everything bakes at once.

2   **3-ounce packages ramen noodles, seasoning packets discarded**
16 **ounces frozen Asian-style mixed vegetables**
1¼ **cups fat-free, low-sodium chicken broth**
4   **boneless, skinless chicken breast halves (about 4 ounces each), all visible fat discarded**
½   **cup bottled Chinese plum sauce**
1   **teaspoon grated lemon zest**
1   **tablespoon fresh lemon juice**
1   **tablespoon grated peeled gingerroot**
1   **teaspoon soy sauce (lowest sodium available)**

Preheat the oven to 350°F.

Break up the noodles over a 13 × 9 × 2-inch glass baking dish or shallow 3-quart glass casserole dish. Spread them in a single layer. Spread the vegetables over the noodles. Pour the broth over all. Arrange the chicken on top.

In a small bowl, stir together the remaining ingredients. Spoon over the chicken.

Bake, covered, for 50 minutes, or until the chicken is no longer pink in the center and the vegetables and noodles are tender.

quick cassoulet

SERVES 5
1 cup per serving

PREPARATION TIME
15 minutes

COOKING TIME
15 to 17 minutes

PER SERVING
Calories 323
Total Fat 4.0 g
  Saturated Fat 0.5 g
  Trans Fat 0.0 g
  Polyunsaturated Fat 1.0 g
  Monounsaturated Fat 1.5 g
Cholesterol 41 mg
Sodium 397 mg
Carbohydrates 50 g
  Fiber 13 g
  Sugars 17 g
Protein 23 g
Dietary Exchanges
  2 starch, 2 vegetable,
  ½ other carbohydrate,
  2 very lean meat

A typical French cassoulet—a hearty mixture of meat, beans, and vegetables—can take up to three days of slow cooking so the flavors blend. This version uses canned beans as a shortcut (dinner will be ready in a half-hour) and adds pizzazz with brown sugar, molasses, allspice, and dry mustard.

Cooking spray

2 or 3 medium carrots, chopped

2 medium ribs of celery, chopped

1 small onion, chopped

1 teaspoon bottled minced garlic or 2 medium garlic cloves, minced

8 ounces boneless, skinless chicken breasts, all visible fat discarded, cut into bite-size pieces

2 15.5-ounce cans no-salt-added Great Northern beans, rinsed and drained

1 8-ounce can no-salt-added tomato sauce

1 cup chopped lower-sodium, low-fat ham

2 tablespoons firmly packed light or dark brown sugar

2 tablespoons molasses (dark preferred)

¼ teaspoon ground allspice

¼ teaspoon dry mustard

¼ teaspoon pepper

Lightly spray a large skillet with cooking spray. Cook the carrots, celery, onion, and garlic over medium-high heat for 7 minutes, or until tender, stirring frequently.

Stir in the chicken. Cook for 2 to 3 minutes, or until just tender, stirring frequently.

Stir in the remaining ingredients. Reduce the heat to medium low. Cook for 5 minutes, or until the chicken is no longer pink in the center and the cassoulet is heated through, stirring occasionally.

chicken jambalaya

SERVES 4
2 cups per serving

PREPARATION TIME
15 to 20 minutes

COOKING TIME
25 minutes

PER SERVING
Calories 285
Total Fat 4.0 g
 Saturated Fat 1.0 g
 Trans Fat 0.0 g
 Polyunsaturated Fat 0.5 g
 Monounsaturated Fat 1.0 g
Cholesterol 66 mg
Sodium 571 mg
Carbohydrates 34 g
 Fiber 5 g
 Sugars 11 g
Protein 26 g
Dietary Exchanges
 1 starch, 4 vegetable,
 2½ very lean meat

The Cajuns perfected the spicy chicken-and-rice dish known as jambalaya. With this recipe, you can now enjoy a quick and healthful version at home.

Cooking spray
1 medium green bell pepper, chopped
1 medium red bell pepper, chopped
1 medium rib of celery, chopped
1 medium onion, chopped
1½ teaspoons bottled minced garlic or 3 medium garlic cloves, minced
2 14.5-ounce cans no-salt-added diced tomatoes, undrained
1 cup uncooked instant brown rice
1 teaspoon dried thyme, crumbled
1 teaspoon pepper
¼ teaspoon salt
¼ teaspoon cayenne
12 ounces boneless, skinless chicken breasts, all visible fat discarded, cut into bite-size pieces
3 ounces Canadian bacon, chopped

Lightly spray a Dutch oven with cooking spray. Cook the bell peppers, celery, onion, and garlic over medium-high heat for 7 minutes, or until tender, stirring frequently.

Stir in the tomatoes with liquid, rice, thyme, pepper, salt, and cayenne. Stir in the chicken and Canadian bacon. Increase the heat to high and bring to a boil. Reduce the heat and simmer, covered, for 15 minutes, or until the chicken is no longer pink in the center, the rice is tender, and the liquid is absorbed.

chicken tenders

IN CREAMY HERB SAUCE

SERVES 4
3 ounces chicken and
2 tablespoons sauce
per serving

PREPARATION TIME
10 minutes

COOKING TIME
16 to 17 minutes

PER SERVING
Calories 173
Total Fat 5.0 g
  Saturated Fat 1.0 g
  Trans Fat 0.0 g
  Polyunsaturated Fat 0.5 g
  Monounsaturated Fat 2.5 g
Cholesterol 73 mg
Sodium 225 mg
Carbohydrates 3 g
  Fiber 0 g
  Sugars 1 g
Protein 27 g
Dietary Exchanges
  3 lean meat

This dish fills the bill when a light, fresh entrée is what you want. Save some room for Sherbet Parfaits (page 253) to end your meal on a sweet note.

2 **teaspoons olive oil**
1 **pound chicken breast tenders, all visible fat discarded**
½ **cup fat-free plain Greek yogurt**
1 **teaspoon all-purpose flour**
⅛ **teaspoon salt**
⅛ **teaspoon cayenne**
½ **cup fat-free, low-sodium chicken broth**
1 **medium shallot, finely chopped**
½ **teaspoon bottled minced garlic or 1 medium garlic clove, minced**
¼ **cup snipped fresh parsley, oregano, dillweed, or other fresh herb**

In a large nonstick skillet, heat the oil over medium-high heat, swirling to coat the bottom. Cook the chicken for 4 minutes. Turn over. Cook for 2 to 3 minutes, or until no longer pink in the center. Transfer to a large plate. Cover to keep warm.

Meanwhile, in a small bowl, whisk together the yogurt, flour, salt, and cayenne. Set aside.

In the same skillet, stir together the broth, shallot, and garlic. Bring to a boil, still over medium high. Boil gently for about 5 minutes, or until most of the liquid is evaporated.

Reduce the heat to low. Whisk in the yogurt mixture and parsley. Cook for 1 minute, whisking constantly.

Return the chicken to the skillet, stirring to coat with the sauce.

COOK'S TIP
Adding flour helps stabilize the yogurt so it doesn't curdle from the heat of the skillet.

chicken
WITH BROCCOLI AND BULGUR

SERVES 4
1½ cups per serving

PREPARATION TIME
10 minutes

COOKING TIME
12 to 16 minutes

PER SERVING
Calories 210
Total Fat 3.0 g
  Saturated Fat 0.5 g
  Trans Fat 0.0 g
  Polyunsaturated Fat 0.5 g
  Monounsaturated Fat 0.5 g
Cholesterol 54 mg
Sodium 271 mg
Carbohydrates 25 g
  Fiber 6 g
  Sugars 1 g
Protein 23 g
Dietary Exchanges
  1½ starch, 1 vegetable,
  2½ very lean meat

This one-dish meal, prepared in one skillet on your stovetop, get its flavor from chicken bouillon granules, lemon zest, and sage and its nutrition from lean chicken, bulgur, and broccoli.

Cooking spray
12 ounces boneless, skinless chicken breasts, all visible fat discarded, cut into bite-size pieces
1 teaspoon bottled minced garlic or 2 medium garlic cloves, minced
1½ cups water
¾ cup uncooked instant, or fine-grain, bulgur
1 teaspoon very low sodium chicken bouillon granules
1 teaspoon grated lemon zest
¼ teaspoon dried sage
¼ teaspoon salt
8 ounces broccoli florets, broken into bite-size pieces (about 3 cups)
Pepper to taste (optional)

Lightly spray a large skillet with cooking spray. Heat over medium-high heat. Cook the chicken and garlic for 2 to 3 minutes, turning the chicken once halfway through.

Stir in the water, bulgur, bouillon granules, lemon zest, sage, and salt. Arrange the broccoli on top. Increase the heat to high and bring to a boil. Reduce the heat and simmer, covered, for 7 to 10 minutes, or until the chicken is no longer pink in the center and the broccoli and bulgur are tender. Sprinkle with the pepper.

chicken and black bean tacos

SERVES 6
2 tacos per serving

PREPARATION TIME
10 minutes

COOKING TIME
10 minutes

PER SERVING
Calories 221
Total Fat 3.0 g
  Saturated Fat 0.5 g
  Trans Fat 0.0 g
  Polyunsaturated Fat 0.5 g
  Monounsaturated Fat 1.0 g
Cholesterol 48 mg
Sodium 244 mg
Carbohydrates 27 g
  Fiber 5 g
  Sugars 3 g
Protein 22 g
Dietary Exchanges
  2 starch, 2½ very lean meat

WITH TOPPINGS

Calories 236
Total Fat 3.5 g
  Saturated Fat 1.0 g
  Trans Fat 0.0 g
  Polyunsaturated Fat 0.5 g
  Monounsaturated Fat 1.0 g
Cholesterol 49 mg
Sodium 276 mg
Carbohydrates 28 g
  Fiber 5 g
  Sugars 4 g
Protein 23 g
Dietary Exchanges
  2 starch, 2½ very lean meat

Certain to become a family favorite, these soft tacos are made with ground chicken, black beans, fresh cilantro, and typical Tex-Mex seasonings. Be sure to have a lot of napkins handy for these messy-but-good tacos.

12 6-inch corn tortillas

FILLING

  1 pound ground skinless chicken breast
  ½ cup chopped onion
  ½ teaspoon bottled minced garlic or 1 medium garlic clove, minced
  1 15.5-ounce can no-salt-added black beans, undrained
  ¼ cup snipped fresh cilantro or parsley
  1 tablespoon chili powder
  ½ teaspoon ground cumin
  ¼ teaspoon salt
  ¼ teaspoon pepper

TOPPINGS (OPTIONAL)

  ¼ cup chopped tomatoes
  ¼ cup shredded lettuce
  ¼ cup shredded low-fat Cheddar cheese
  ½ cup plus 2 tablespoons Chunky Salsa (page 32) or commercial salsa (lowest sodium available)

Preheat the oven to 250°F. Wrap the tortillas in aluminum foil. Put in the oven while preparing the chicken mixture.

In a large skillet, cook the chicken, onion, and garlic over medium-high heat for 5 minutes, or until the chicken is no longer pink in the center, stirring occasionally to turn and break up the chicken.

Stir in the remaining filling ingredients. Cook for 5 minutes, or until heated through.

Place 2 tortillas on each plate. Spoon the chicken mixture over half of each tortilla. Add the toppings. Fold the other half of each tortilla over the filling.

grilled chicken burgers

SERVES 6
1 burger per serving

PREPARATION TIME
8 to 10 minutes

COOKING TIME
8 to 10 minutes

PER SERVING

Calories 136
Total Fat 2.5 g
  Saturated Fat 0.5 g
  Trans Fat 0.0 g
  Polyunsaturated Fat 0.5 g
  Monounsaturated Fat 0.5 g
Cholesterol 48 mg
Sodium 241 mg
Carbohydrates 10 g
  Fiber 1 g
  Sugars 3 g
Protein 17 g
Dietary Exchanges
  ½ starch, 2 very lean meat

Serve these sizzling burgers right off the grill or tucked with lettuce and tomatoes inside pita pockets.

Cooking spray
1 **pound ground skinless chicken breast**
½ **cup plain dry bread crumbs (lowest sodium available)**
2 **medium green onions, chopped**
2 **tablespoons barbecue sauce (lowest sodium available)**
1 **tablespoon fresh lemon juice**
2 **teaspoons Worcestershire sauce (lowest sodium available)**
⅛ **teaspoon salt**

Lightly spray the grill rack or the broiler pan and rack with cooking spray. Preheat the grill on medium high or preheat the broiler.

In a large bowl, using your hands or a spoon, combine all the burger ingredients. Shape into 6 patties about ¼ inch thick.

Grill the patties or broil 3 to 4 inches from the heat for 4 to 5 minutes on each side, or until the patties are no longer pink in the center.

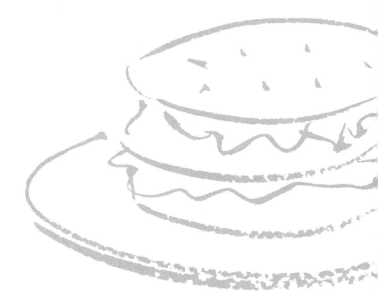

cornmeal chicken muffinwiches

SERVES 6
1 muffinwich per serving

PREPARATION TIME
10 to 12 minutes

COOKING TIME
15 to 20 minutes

PER SERVING

Calories 230
Total Fat 4.5 g
 Saturated Fat 1.0 g
 Trans Fat 0.0 g
 Polyunsaturated Fat 1.0 g
 Monounsaturated Fat 2.0 g
Cholesterol 32 mg
Sodium 419 mg
Carbohydrates 31 g
 Fiber 1 g
 Sugars 9 g
Protein 16 g
Dietary Exchanges
 2 starch, 2 very lean meat

Serve this handy sandwich-in-a-muffin with Double-Tomato Soup (page 45), then freeze any extras (or make a second batch). Pop a frozen muffinwich into a lunch box or brown bag in the morning, and it will be thawed by noon.

Cooking spray
1 8.5-ounce package corn muffin mix
2 large egg whites
⅓ cup fat-free milk
8 ounces coarsely chopped cooked skinless chicken breast (about 2 cups), cooked without salt, all visible fat discarded
4 medium green onions, sliced
¼ teaspoon dried sage

Preheat the oven to 400°F. Lightly spray a standard 6-cup muffin pan with cooking spray or line with paper bake cups. Set aside.

Prepare the muffin mix using the package directions, substituting the egg whites for the egg and the fat-free milk for whole milk. Fold in the chicken, green onions, and sage. Spoon into the muffin cups.

Bake for 15 to 20 minutes, or until a wooden toothpick inserted in the center comes out clean. Transfer the muffins from the muffin pan to a cooling rack. Serve warm or at room temperature. Freeze any extra muffins in an airtight bag for up to two months.

turkey tenderloin

WITH CRANBERRY-JALAPEÑO SAUCE

SERVES 4
3 ounces turkey and
¼ cup sauce per serving

PREPARATION TIME
10 to 12 minutes

COOKING TIME
32 to 42 minutes

STANDING TIME
5 to 10 minutes

PER SERVING
Calories 280
Total Fat 2.0 g
  Saturated Fat 0.5 g
  Trans Fat 0.0 g
  Polyunsaturated Fat 0.5 g
  Monounsaturated Fat 1.0 g
Cholesterol 70 mg
Sodium 77 mg
Carbohydrates 37 g
  Fiber 2 g
  Sugars 24 g
Protein 28 g
Dietary Exchanges
  2½ other carbohydrate,
  3 very lean meat

You can enjoy this combination of turkey and cranberries year-round—no need to wait for Thanksgiving! The small amount of fresh jalapeño provides an underlying hint of heat.

    Cooking spray
  1 **1-pound turkey tenderloin**
  1 **teaspoon canola or corn oil**
  14 **ounces whole-berry cranberry sauce**
  2 **teaspoons grated orange zest**
  1½ **tablespoons snipped fresh cilantro**
  1 **teaspoon minced fresh jalapeño**

Preheat the oven to 400°F.

Lightly spray a large glass baking dish with cooking spray. Put the turkey in the baking dish, tucking the ends of the turkey under for even cooking. Brush the top with the oil.

Roast for 20 minutes.

Meanwhile, in a small saucepan, stir together the cranberry sauce, orange zest, cilantro, and jalapeño. Cook over low heat for 5 minutes, or until heated through, stirring once. Remove from the heat. Spoon 1 cup of the sauce into a small bowl and set aside. You should have about ½ cup sauce left in the pan.

Turn the turkey over. Baste with about half the cranberry sauce from the pan.

Roast for 10 to 20 minutes, or until the turkey registers 160°F on an instant-read thermometer, basting once about halfway through with the remaining sauce in the pan. Transfer the turkey to a cutting board. Let stand for 5 to 10 minutes, or until it is no longer pink in the center and registers 165°F. Thinly slice diagonally across the grain. Serve with the reserved 1 cup sauce spooned on top.

COOK'S TIP
If you can't find a turkey tenderloin about the size called for, you can use two half-pound pieces or four quarter-pound pieces. Arrange them so they make a cylinder, and use kitchen twine to tie the pieces together at about 2-inch intervals.

southwestern turkey stew

SERVES 8
1¼ cups per serving

PREPARATION TIME
13 to 15 minutes

COOKING TIME
28 minutes

OR

MICROWAVE TIME
15 minutes

PER SERVING
Calories 185
Total Fat 1.0 g
  Saturated Fat 0.0 g
  Trans Fat 0.0 g
  Polyunsaturated Fat 0.5 g
  Monounsaturated Fat 0.0 g
Cholesterol 53 mg
Sodium 264 mg
Carbohydrates 20 g
  Fiber 3 g
  Sugars 6 g
Protein 24 g
Dietary Exchanges
  1 starch, 1 vegetable,
  2½ very lean meat

Because it uses a number of highly flavored ingredients, this stew doesn't need long, slow cooking to be delicious.

- ¼ cup all-purpose flour
- ½ teaspoon salt
- ⅛ teaspoon pepper
- 1½ pounds turkey tenderloins, cut into ½-inch cubes
- 2 14.5-ounce cans no-salt-added diced tomatoes, undrained
- 1¼ cups fat-free, low-sodium chicken broth
- 10 ounces frozen whole-kernel corn
- 1 large onion, chopped
- 1 4-ounce can chopped green chiles, drained
- 2 teaspoons bottled minced garlic or 4 medium garlic cloves, minced
- 1½ teaspoons ground cumin
- 1½ teaspoons dried oregano, crumbled
- ¼ cup snipped fresh cilantro

In a large shallow dish, stir together the flour, salt, and pepper. Add the turkey, turning to coat well and gently shaking off any excess. Transfer to a Dutch oven.

Stir in the remaining ingredients except the cilantro. Bring to a boil over high heat. Reduce the heat and simmer, covered, for 25 minutes, or until the turkey is no longer pink in the center, stirring occasionally. Just before serving, stir in the cilantro.

MICROWAVE METHOD

Halve the ingredients listed above (the recipe will serve 4 as a main dish). Prepare the turkey as directed. In a 2-quart microwaveable casserole dish, stir together the turkey and the remaining ingredients except the cilantro. Microwave, covered, on 100 percent power (high) for 15 minutes, or until the turkey is no longer pink in the center, stirring twice. Remove from the microwave. Stir in the cilantro.

roast turkey tenderloin
WITH MASHED SWEET POTATOES AND FRUIT

These delightfully different mashed sweet potatoes go well with turkey, as in this recipe, or try them with pork tenderloin or roasted chicken.

　　Cooking spray
2　pounds turkey tenderloins
½　teaspoon ground coriander
¼　teaspoon pepper and ⅛ teaspoon pepper, divided use
⅛　teaspoon salt and ⅛ teaspoon salt, divided use
2　pounds sweet potatoes, peeled and cut into large chunks
3　medium pears (Bartlett or Bosc preferred) or apples (Golden Delicious, Granny Smith, or Rome Beauty preferred), peeled and cut into large chunks
1　cinnamon stick (about 3 inches long)
1　tablespoon light tub margarine

Preheat the oven to 350°F.

　　Lightly spray a large glass baking dish with cooking spray. Put the turkey in the baking dish, tucking the ends of the turkey under for even cooking. Sprinkle with the coriander, ¼ teaspoon pepper, and ⅛ teaspoon salt.

　　Roast for 35 to 40 minutes, or until the turkey registers 160°F on an instant-read thermometer. Transfer the turkey to a cutting board. Let stand for 5 to 10 minutes, or until it is no longer pink in the center and registers 165°F. Thinly slice diagonally across the grain.

　　Meanwhile, put the sweet potatoes, pears, and cinnamon stick in a Dutch oven. Add enough water to cover. Bring to a boil over high heat. Reduce the heat and simmer, covered, for 20 minutes, or until the sweet potatoes and pears are tender. Drain well. Discard the cinnamon stick.

　　If using an electric hand mixer to beat the potato mixture, leave the mixture in the pan. If using an electric stand mixer, transfer the mixture to a large mixing bowl. Beat on low speed until smooth. Stir in the margarine, remaining and ⅛ teaspoon pepper and remaining ⅛ teaspoon salt. (You can use a potato masher if you prefer.) Serve the potato mixture with the turkey.

turkey medallions

WITH ROSEMARY-MUSHROOM GRAVY

SERVES 4
3 ounces turkey and
2 tablespoons gravy
per serving

PREPARATION TIME
13 minutes

COOKING TIME
22 minutes

PER SERVING
Calories 182
Total Fat 3.0 g
  Saturated Fat 0.5 g
  Trans Fat 0.0 g
  Polyunsaturated Fat 0.5 g
  Monounsaturated Fat 2.0 g
Cholesterol 70 mg
Sodium 215 mg
Carbohydrates 7 g
  Fiber 1 g
  Sugars 3 g
Protein 30 g
Dietary Exchanges
  ½ other carbohydrate,
  3 very lean meat

*Chanterelle mushroom sauce adds a delicate, meaty flavor
and richness to this dish.*

  1 **tablespoon cornstarch**
  ½ **cup fat-free, low-sodium chicken broth**
  ¼ **teaspoon salt**
  ⅛ **teaspoon pepper**
     Cooking spray
  1 **teaspoon olive oil and 1 teaspoon olive oil,
     divided use**
  1 **1-pound turkey tenderloin, all visible fat
     discarded, cut crosswise into ¼-inch slices**
  2 **tablespoons balsamic vinegar**
  1 **teaspoon finely snipped fresh rosemary
     or ¼ teaspoon dried, crushed**
  8 **ounces chanterelle or button mushrooms, sliced
     (about 2½ cups)**
  ¼ **cup chopped shallot or onion**

Put the cornstarch in a small bowl. Add the broth,
stirring to dissolve. Stir in the salt and pepper. Set aside.

  Lightly spray a large skillet with cooking spray. Heat
1 teaspoon oil over medium-high heat, swirling to coat
the bottom. Cook half the turkey medallions in a single
layer for 2 minutes on each side, or until no longer
pink in the center. Transfer to a large plate. Cover to
keep warm. Repeat with the remaining 1 teaspoon oil
and remaining turkey medallions. Remove the skillet
from the heat.

  Add the vinegar and rosemary to the skillet, scraping
to dislodge any browned bits. Return to the heat. Stir
in the mushrooms and shallot. Cook over medium heat
for 5 minutes, or until the mushrooms are soft, stirring
occasionally.

  Stir the cornstarch mixture. Pour into the mushroom
mixture. Cook for 5 minutes, or until thickened and
bubbly, stirring frequently. Serve the sauce with the
turkey.

turkey and artichoke fettuccine

SERVES 4
1½ cups per serving

PREPARATION TIME
8 minutes

COOKING TIME
15 minutes

PER SERVING

Calories 483
Total Fat 5.0 g
  Saturated Fat 2.0 g
  Trans Fat 0.0 g
  Polyunsaturated Fat 1.0 g
  Monounsaturated Fat 1.5 g
Cholesterol 81 mg
Sodium 515 mg
Carbohydrates 61 g
  Fiber 11 g
  Sugars 13 g
Protein 48 g
Dietary Exchanges
  3 starch, 1 vegetable,
  1 fat-free milk,
  3½ very lean meat

Artichoke hearts add a special touch to this all-in-one combination. It's perfect if you want an elegant dinner but don't have lots of time to spend in the kitchen.

8   ounces dried whole-grain fettuccine
9   ounces frozen artichoke hearts or frozen broccoli florets
    Cooking spray
1   pound turkey tenderloin, all visible fat discarded, cut into bite-size pieces
½   teaspoon bottled minced garlic or 1 medium garlic clove, minced
1   tablespoon all-purpose flour
1   12-ounce can fat-free evaporated milk
¼   teaspoon salt
¼   teaspoon dried marjoram or basil, crumbled
⅛   teaspoon pepper
⅛   teaspoon ground nutmeg (optional)
½   cup shredded or grated Parmesan cheese

In a soup pot, prepare the pasta using the package directions, omitting the salt. During the last 5 minutes of cooking, stir in the artichokes. Drain well in a colander. Halve any large artichoke hearts. Return to the pan. Cover to keep warm.

Meanwhile, lightly spray a large skillet with cooking spray. Heat over medium-high heat. Cook the turkey and garlic for 3 minutes, or until the turkey is no longer pink in the center, stirring occasionally.

Stir in the flour. Stir in the remaining ingredients except the Parmesan. Cook for 6 minutes, or until thickened and bubbly, stirring constantly.

Add the turkey mixture and Parmesan to the pasta, tossing to coat.

velvet turkey and herbs

SERVES 4

2/3 cup per serving

PREPARATION TIME

10 minutes

COOKING TIME

9 to 10 minutes

PER SERVING

Calories 224
Total Fat 1.0 g
  Saturated Fat 0.5 g
  Trans Fat 0.0 g
  Polyunsaturated Fat 0.0 g
  Monounsaturated Fat 0.0 g
Cholesterol 74 mg
Sodium 240 mg
Carbohydrates 16 g
  Fiber 0 g
  Sugars 11 g
Protein 36 g
Dietary Exchanges
  1 fat-free milk,
  ½ other carbohydrate,
  3 very lean meat

A smooth-as-velvet sauce with a trio of fresh herbs added makes this an entrée not to be missed. Serve it with whole-wheat orzo and Swiss chard.

Cooking spray
1 pound turkey tenderloin, all visible fat discarded, cut into bite-size pieces
¼ cup chopped shallot or onion
½ teaspoon bottled minced garlic or 1 medium garlic clove, minced
2 tablespoons all-purpose flour
1 12-ounce can fat-free evaporated milk
1 tablespoon snipped fresh oregano or ½ teaspoon dried, crumbled
1 tablespoon snipped fresh parsley
1 teaspoon snipped fresh basil or ¼ teaspoon dried, crumbled
⅛ teaspoon salt

Lightly spray a large skillet with cooking spray. Heat over medium-high heat. Cook the turkey, shallot, and garlic for 3 to 4 minutes, or until the turkey is no longer pink in the center, stirring occasionally.

Stir in the flour. Stir in the remaining ingredients. Cook for 4 minutes, or until thickened and bubbly, stirring constantly.

currant turkey
WITH CAPERS

SERVES 4
3 ounces turkey and
2 tablespoons sauce
per serving

PREPARATION TIME
8 minutes

COOKING TIME
15 minutes

PER SERVING
Calories 188
Total Fat 1.0 g
  Saturated Fat 0.5 g
  Trans Fat 0.0 g
  Polyunsaturated Fat 0.5 g
  Monounsaturated Fat 0.0 g
Cholesterol 70 mg
Sodium 268 mg
Carbohydrates 10 g
  Fiber 1 g
  Sugars 6 g
Protein 28 g
Dietary Exchanges
  ½ other carbohydrate,
  3 very lean meat

The sweetness of currants and the saltiness of capers come together tastefully in an unusual sauce that tops lightly browned slices of turkey breast.

Cooking spray
1 pound turkey cutlets, all visible fat discarded
½ cup dry white wine and 2 tablespoons dry white wine (regular or nonalcoholic), divided use
¼ cup dried currants or raisins
2 tablespoons chopped onion
1 tablespoon capers, drained and chopped
½ teaspoon bottled minced garlic or 1 medium garlic clove, minced
¼ teaspoon salt
¼ teaspoon ground cinnamon
1 tablespoon cornstarch

Lightly spray a large skillet with cooking spray. Heat over medium-high heat. Cook half the turkey for 1 minute on each side, or until browned (the turkey will not be done at this point). Transfer to a large plate. Repeat with the remaining turkey. Set aside.

Slowly pour ½ cup wine into the skillet, scraping to dislodge any browned bits. Stir in the currants, onion, capers, garlic, salt, and cinnamon. Bring to a boil over medium-high heat. Return the turkey to the skillet. Reduce the heat and simmer, covered, for 2 minutes, or until the turkey is no longer pink in the center. Transfer the turkey to a separate large plate, leaving the sauce in the skillet. Cover the plate to keep warm.

Put the cornstarch in a small bowl. Add the remaining 2 tablespoons wine, whisking to dissolve. Whisk into the wine mixture in the skillet. Cook for 5 minutes, or until thickened and bubbly, whisking constantly. Serve over the turkey.

fresh herb turkey loaf

SERVES 6
1 slice per serving

PREPARATION TIME
12 to 15 minutes

COOKING TIME
40 to 45 minutes

STANDING TIME
5 minutes

MICROWAVE TIME
40 to 45 seconds

PER SERVING
Calories 159
Total Fat 1.5 g
  Saturated Fat 0.5 g
  Trans Fat 0.0 g
  Polyunsaturated Fat 0.5 g
  Monounsaturated Fat 0.5 g
Cholesterol 47 mg
Sodium 260 mg
Carbohydrates 13 g
  Fiber 2 g
  Sugars 2 g
Protein 23 g
Dietary Exchanges
  ½ starch, 1 vegetable,
  2½ very lean meat

It's the use of fresh parsley and basil or oregano that sets this turkey loaf apart.

Cooking spray
1 pound ground skinless turkey breast
1 cup uncooked rolled oats
½ medium red bell pepper, chopped
1 small to medium rib of celery, finely chopped
¼ cup chopped shallot or onion
2 large egg whites
2 tablespoons snipped fresh Italian (flat-leaf) parsley and 1 teaspoon snipped fresh Italian (flat-leaf) parsley, divided use
2 tablespoons snipped fresh basil or oregano and 1 teaspoon snipped fresh basil or oregano, divided use
½ teaspoon salt
¼ teaspoon pepper
½ cup no-salt-added tomato sauce

Preheat the oven to 350°F. Lightly spray a 9 × 5 × 3-inch loaf pan with cooking spray.

In a medium bowl, using your hands or a spoon, combine the turkey, oats, bell pepper, celery, shallot, egg whites, 2 tablespoons parsley, 2 tablespoons basil, salt, and pepper. Transfer to the pan, lightly smoothing the top.

Bake for 40 to 45 minutes, or until the loaf registers 165°F on an instant-read thermometer. Using paper towels, pat dry any moisture that has risen to the top. Let stand at room temperature for 5 minutes to finish cooking. Cut the loaf into 6 slices. Transfer to plates.

Pour the tomato sauce into a small microwaveable bowl. Microwave, covered, on 100 percent power (high) for 40 to 45 seconds, or until hot. Pour over the turkey loaf slices. Sprinkle with the remaining 1 teaspoon parsley and remaining 1 teaspoon basil.

meats

molasses-marinated tenderloin

SERVES 4
3 ounces beef and
1½ tablespoons sauce
per serving

PREPARATION TIME
5 minutes

MARINATING TIME
24 hours

COOKING TIME
11 to 13 minutes

PER SERVING
Calories 239
Total Fat 5.0 g
  Saturated Fat 2.5 g
  Trans Fat 0.0 g
  Polyunsaturated Fat 0.5 g
  Monounsaturated Fat 2.5 g
Cholesterol 53 mg
Sodium 208 mg
Carbohydrates 23 g
  Fiber 0 g
  Sugars 17 g
Protein 24 g
Dietary Exchanges
  1½ other carbohydrate,
  3 lean meat

Molasses gives this marinade a deliciously rich flavor. Because the molasses mixture tends to caramelize during cooking, be sure to use a nonstick skillet for easier cleanup.

⅓ **cup light molasses**
 1 **medium shallot, chopped**
 2 **tablespoons balsamic vinegar or red wine vinegar**
½ **teaspoon dried thyme, crumbled**
¼ **teaspoon salt**
¼ **teaspoon pepper**
 1 **1-pound beef tenderloin, all visible fat discarded**

In a large shallow glass dish, stir together the molasses, shallot, vinegar, thyme, salt, and pepper. Add the beef, turning to coat. Cover and refrigerate for about 24 hours, turning occasionally.

About 15 minutes before serving time, transfer the beef to a cutting board, reserving the marinade. Cut the beef crosswise into 4 slices.

Heat a large nonstick skillet over medium-high heat. Cook the beef for 3 minutes. Turn over. Cook for 3 to 5 minutes, or to the desired doneness. Transfer to a large plate. Cover to keep warm.

Pour the marinade into the same skillet. Cook, still over medium-high heat, for 3 minutes, or until the marinade just begins to boil. Spoon over the beef.

beef tenderloin
ON HERBED WHITE BEANS

SERVES 4
3 ounces beef and
½ cup beans
per serving

PREPARATION TIME
10 minutes

COOKING TIME
9 minutes

PER SERVING
Calories 261
Total Fat 6.5 g
  Saturated Fat 2.5 g
  Trans Fat 0.0 g
  Polyunsaturated Fat 0.5 g
  Monounsaturated Fat 3.5 g
Cholesterol 53 mg
Sodium 354 mg
Carbohydrates 19 g
  Fiber 6 g
  Sugars 1 g
Protein 30 g
Dietary Exchanges
  1½ starch, 3½ lean meat

*Although you need only a small amount of fresh herbs
for this dish, try using a combination of your favorites or
of what you have on hand. Some possibilities are basil,
oregano, marjoram, thyme, chives, and dillweed.*

  Pepper to taste
1 **1-pound beef tenderloin, all visible fat discarded,
  cut crosswise into 4 slices**
  Cooking spray
1 **teaspoon olive oil**
½ **cup chopped red onion**
½ **teaspoon bottled minced garlic or 1 medium garlic
  clove, minced**
1 **15.5-ounce can no-salt-added navy beans, about
  1 inch of liquid discarded**
1 **tablespoon chopped fresh herbs or 1 teaspoon
  dried herbs, crumbled, and (optional) fresh herbs
  for garnish, divided use**
½ **teaspoon salt**

Sprinkle the pepper over both sides of the beef. Using
your fingertips, gently press the pepper so it adheres to
the beef.

Lightly spray a large skillet with cooking spray. Heat
over medium-high heat. Cook the beef for 3 minutes.
Turn over. Cook for 3 to 5 minutes, or to the desired
doneness.

Meanwhile, lightly spray a small saucepan with
cooking spray. Heat the oil over medium-high heat,
swirling to coat the bottom. Cook the onion and
garlic for 3 minutes, or until the onion is soft, stirring
frequently.

Stir in the beans with the remaining liquid, the herbs,
and salt. Reduce the heat to low. Cook for 5 minutes, or
until heated through. Spoon onto plates. Top with the
beef. Garnish with the remaining fresh herbs.

flank steak

WITH BLUEBERRY-POMEGRANATE SAUCE

SERVES 4
3 ounces beef and
2 tablespoons sauce
per serving

PREPARATION TIME
9 minutes

COOKING TIME
21 to 25 minutes

PER SERVING
Calories 185
Total Fat 6.5 g
   Saturated Fat 3.0 g
   Trans Fat 0.0 g
   Polyunsaturated Fat 0.5 g
   Monounsaturated Fat 3.0 g
Cholesterol 48 mg
Sodium 207 mg
Carbohydrates 6 g
   Fiber 1 g
   Sugars 4 g
Protein 24 g
Dietary Exchanges
   ½ fruit, 3 lean meat

Reducing beef broth with blueberry-pomegranate juice creates a sauce with deep flavor undertones. If you like your sauce a bit less sweet, you can omit the maple syrup.

¼   **teaspoon pepper**
¼   **teaspoon salt**
1   **1-pound flank steak, cut about ¾ inch thick, all visible fat discarded**
   Cooking spray
½   **cup fresh or frozen blueberries (wild preferred)**
½   **cup fat-free, no-salt-added beef broth**
¼   **cup frozen pomegranate juice concentrate (blueberry-pomegranate preferred) or grape juice concentrate, thawed**
½   **teaspoon bottled minced garlic or 1 medium garlic clove, minced**
2   **tablespoons snipped fresh parsley**
1   **tablespoon maple syrup (optional)**
2   **teaspoons balsamic vinegar**

Sprinkle the pepper and salt over both sides of the beef. Using your fingertips, gently press the seasonings so they adhere to the beef.

Lightly spray a large skillet with cooking spray. Heat over medium heat. Cook the beef for 10 to 12 minutes, or until rare (the beef won't be done at this point), turning once halfway through. Transfer the beef to a cutting board.

In the same skillet, stir together the blueberries, broth, pomegranate juice, and garlic, scraping the skillet to dislodge any browned bits. Bring to a boil over medium-high heat. Boil for 5 to 6 minutes, or until the liquid is reduced to about ⅓ cup.

While the sauce boils, thinly slice the steak across the grain. Set aside.

Stir the parsley, maple syrup, and vinegar into the sauce. Return the beef to the skillet, turning to coat with the sauce. Cook for 1 to 2 minutes, or until the beef is heated through and cooked to the desired doneness.

COOK'S TIP ON WILD BLUEBERRIES

Wild blueberries are more flavorful than "regular" blueberries. If you want a big flavor punch and can't find wild blueberries, you can substitute dried blueberries, but use only half as much as called for. Keep in mind, though, that the dried fruit contains much more sugar—and therefore more calories. Wild blueberries can be found in local grocery stores, but you may have difficulty finding the fresh variety if you live outside New England. Maine produces nearly all the country's wild blueberries and their season is short. If you can't find them in the produce department, check the frozen aisle.

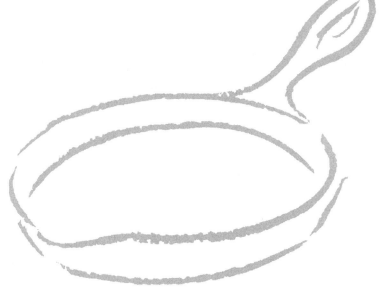

pepper-rubbed beef

WITH MUSHROOM SAUCE

SERVES 4
3 ounces beef and
¼ cup sauce
per serving

PREPARATION TIME
7 minutes

COOKING TIME
10 minutes

PER SERVING
Calories 235
Total Fat 7.0 g
  Saturated Fat 3.0 g
  Trans Fat 0.0 g
  Polyunsaturated Fat 0.5 g
  Monounsaturated Fat 3.5 g
Cholesterol 51 mg
Sodium 316 mg
Carbohydrates 12 g
  Fiber 1 g
  Sugars 9 g
Protein 30 g
Dietary Exchanges
  ½ fat-free milk,
  ½ other carbohydrate,
  3 lean meat

A creamy mushroom sauce spiked with Dijon mustard dresses up lean flank steak.

　　Cooking spray
2　teaspoons pepper (coarsely ground preferred)
¼　teaspoon salt
1　1-pound flank steak, all visible fat discarded
4　ounces presliced button mushrooms (about 1¼ cups)
2　medium green onions, sliced
½　teaspoon bottled minced garlic or 1 medium garlic clove, minced
1　tablespoon all-purpose flour
2　teaspoons Dijon mustard (lowest sodium available)
1　cup fat-free evaporated milk

Preheat the broiler. Lightly spray the broiler pan and rack with cooking spray. Set aside.

　　Sprinkle the pepper and salt on both sides of the beef. Using your fingertips, gently press the seasonings so they adhere to the beef.

　　Broil about 4 inches from the heat for 3 to 5 minutes on each side, or to the desired doneness. Transfer to a cutting board. Thinly slice the beef diagonally across the grain.

　　Meanwhile, lightly spray a medium saucepan with cooking spray. Cook the mushrooms, green onions, and garlic over medium heat for 5 minutes, or until the mushrooms are just soft.

　　Stir in the flour. Add the mustard. Pour in the milk all at once. Cook for 5 minutes, or until thickened to the desired consistency, stirring constantly. Spoon over the beef.

grilled sirloin steak

WITH LEMONY HORSERADISH SAUCE

SERVES 4
3 ounces beef and
2½ tablespoons sauce
per serving

PREPARATION TIME
7 minutes

COOKING TIME
8 to 10 minutes

PER SERVING
Calories 213
Total Fat 9.0 g
  Saturated Fat 2.0 g
  Trans Fat 0.0 g
  Polyunsaturated Fat 3.5 g
  Monounsaturated Fat 3.0 g
Cholesterol 66 mg
Sodium 265 mg
Carbohydrates 6 g
  Fiber 0 g
  Sugars 2 g
Protein 25 g
Dietary Exchanges
  ½ other carbohydrate,
  3 lean meat

Top the steak with this spicy sauce. It's also good on lean grilled burgers or steamed red potatoes. Since you'll have a heated grill for your entrée, why not fix Grilled Peaches with Almond Liqueur (page 251) for dessert?

   Cooking spray
SAUCE
   ⅓ cup fat-free sour cream
   ⅓ cup light mayonnaise
   2 tablespoons bottled white horseradish, drained
   ½ teaspoon grated lemon zest
   1 teaspoon fresh lemon juice

   1 pound boneless top sirloin steak, all visible fat
      discarded, cut into 4 pieces

Lightly spray the grill rack with cooking spray. Preheat on medium high.

   In a small bowl, whisk together the sauce ingredients. Set aside or cover and refrigerate until serving time.

   Grill the beef for 4 to 5 minutes on each side, or to the desired doneness. Serve topped with the sauce.

ginger beef and broccoli stir-fry

SERVES 4
1 cup beef and
vegetables per serving

PREPARATION TIME
15 minutes

COOKING TIME
10 to 13 minutes

PER SERVING

Calories 214
Total Fat 7.5 g
  Saturated Fat 2.0 g
  Trans Fat 0.0 g
  Polyunsaturated Fat 1.0 g
  Monounsaturated Fat 4.0 g
Cholesterol 60 mg
Sodium 296 mg
Carbohydrates 8 g
  Fiber 2 g
  Sugars 2 g
Protein 29 g
Dietary Exchanges
  2 vegetable, 3 lean meat

Grated gingerroot adds a spicy bite to this family-pleasing stir-fry. Serve it with soba noodles or whole-grain vermicelli on the side.

⅓ **cup fat-free, low-sodium chicken broth**

2 **tablespoons soy sauce (lowest sodium available)**

2 **tablespoons water and 1 to 2 tablespoons water (as needed), divided use**

2 **teaspoons cornstarch**

2 **teaspoons grated peeled gingerroot**

½ **teaspoon bottled minced garlic or 1 medium garlic clove, minced**

¼ **teaspoon toasted sesame oil**

⅛ **teaspoon crushed red pepper flakes**

1 **teaspoon canola or corn oil and 1 teaspoon canola or corn oil, divided use**

1 **pound boneless top sirloin steak, all visible fat discarded, cut across the grain into ¼-inch strips**

12 **ounces broccoli florets, broken into 1-inch pieces (about 4½ cups)**

2 **medium green onions, thinly sliced (optional)**

In a small bowl, combine the broth, soy sauce, 2 tablespoons water, cornstarch, gingerroot, garlic, sesame oil, and red pepper flakes, whisking until the cornstarch is dissolved. Set aside.

In a large nonstick skillet, heat 1 teaspoon canola oil over medium-high heat, swirling to coat the bottom. Cook half the beef for 2 to 3 minutes, or until browned, stirring and turning constantly. Transfer to a medium plate. Repeat with the remaining beef (no additional oil needed). Set all the beef aside.

Heat the remaining 1 teaspoon canola oil in the same skillet, swirling to coat the bottom. Cook the broccoli for 2 to 3 minutes, or until tender-crisp, stirring frequently. If the mixture becomes too dry, add the remaining 1 to 2 tablespoons water as needed.

Stir the beef into the broccoli. Stir the broth mixture, then stir it into the broccoli. Cook for 1 to 2 minutes, or until the beef is heated through and the broth mixture is thickened. Sprinkle with the green onions.

COOK'S TIP ON TOASTED SESAME OIL

Toasted sesame oil is integral to Asian cuisine. Just a small amount infuses an entire dish with sesame flavor. Since you need to use only a little bit for each recipe, a bottle of sesame oil can last a long time. Store it in the refrigerator to prolong its freshness.

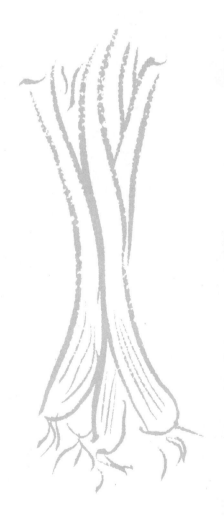

sliced sirloin
WITH LEEK SAUCE

SERVES 4
3 ounces beef and
¼ cup sauce
per serving

PREPARATION TIME
8 to 10 minutes

COOKING TIME
25 to 27 minutes

PER SERVING
Calories 171
Total Fat 4.5 g
  Saturated Fat 2.0 g
  Trans Fat 0.0 g
  Polyunsaturated Fat 0.5 g
  Monounsaturated Fat 2.0 g
Cholesterol 56 mg
Sodium 343 mg
Carbohydrates 4 g
  Fiber 0 g
  Sugars 1 g
Protein 24 g
Dietary Exchanges
  ½ other carbohydrate,
  3 lean meat

You'll love the robust leek sauce that tops this succulent sirloin. Serve the steak with Skillet-Roasted Bell Pepper, Zucchini, and Vermicelli Soup (page 43) and a salad of fresh fruit.

  Cooking spray
 1 **1-pound boneless top sirloin steak, about 1½ inches thick, all visible fat discarded**
 ¾ **cup water and 2 tablespoons water, divided use**
 ¼ **cup dry red wine (regular or nonalcoholic)**
 ½ **cup sliced leeks (white and light green parts only)**
 ½ **teaspoon very low sodium beef bouillon granules**
 ½ **teaspoon bottled minced garlic or 1 medium garlic clove, minced**
 ½ **teaspoon salt**
 1 **tablespoon plus 1 teaspoon all-purpose flour**

Lightly spray a large skillet with cooking spray. Heat over medium-high heat. Cook the beef for 8 minutes on each side, or to the desired doneness. Transfer to a plate. Cover to keep warm.

  In the same skillet, stir together ¾ cup water, the wine, leeks, bouillon granules, garlic, and salt. Bring to a simmer, still over medium high. Reduce the heat and simmer, covered, for 3 minutes.

  Meanwhile, in a small bowl, whisk together the flour and remaining 2 tablespoons water. Whisk into the sauce. Cook for 3 minutes, or until the desired consistency, whisking constantly.

  Cut the beef crosswise into ½-inch slices. Serve topped with the sauce.

COOK'S TIP ON LEEKS
Leeks look like overgrown green onions and have a mild onion flavor. Discard the shaggy root ends and the tough green leaves. The bulbs and light green parts of the leaves that remain are the parts you cook. Be sure to rinse leeks thoroughly to remove the sandy grit that collects between the tight leaves.

steak

WITH SUN-DRIED TOMATOES

SERVES 4

3 ounces beef per serving

PREPARATION TIME

15 minutes

COOKING TIME

12 to 14 minutes

PER SERVING

Calories 156
Total Fat 5.0 g
  Saturated Fat 2.0 g
  Trans Fat 0.0 g
  Polyunsaturated Fat 0.5 g
  Monounsaturated Fat 2.5 g
Cholesterol 56 mg
Sodium 211 mg
Carbohydrates 3 g
  Fiber 1 g
  Sugars 1 g
Protein 24 g
Dietary Exchanges
  3 lean meat

An assertive mixture of sun-dried tomatoes, carrot, green onion, and fresh basil fills pockets cut in pieces of sirloin steak.

4   sun-dried tomatoes, packed in oil, drained, patted dry, and coarsely chopped
¼   to ½ cup preshredded carrot
1   medium green onion, sliced
2   teaspoons chopped fresh basil or ½ teaspoon dried, crumbled
¼   teaspoon salt
    Cooking spray
1   1-pound boneless top sirloin steak, about 1 inch thick, all visible fat discarded
1   teaspoon bottled minced garlic or 2 medium garlic cloves, minced

In a small bowl, stir together the tomatoes, carrot, green onion, basil, and salt. Set aside.

Preheat the broiler. Lightly spray the broiler pan and rack with cooking spray.

Cut the beef in half crosswise. Cut a large slit width-wise in each half (*almost* all the way through) to form a deep pocket. Spoon the tomato mixture into the pockets. Secure the openings with wooden toothpicks. Sprinkle the garlic over the top of the beef.

Broil about 4 inches from the heat for 6 minutes. Turn over. Broil for 6 to 8 minutes, or to the desired doneness. Transfer the beef to a cutting board. Discard the toothpicks. Cut each piece of beef in half.

sirloin
WITH ORANGE-CORIANDER GLAZE

SERVES 4
3 ounces beef per serving

PREPARATION TIME
5 minutes

CHILLING TIME
10 minutes

COOKING TIME
16 to 18 minutes

PER SERVING
Calories 148
Total Fat 4.5 g
  Saturated Fat 2.0 g
  Trans Fat 0.0 g
  Polyunsaturated Fat 0.0 g
  Monounsaturated Fat 2.0 g
Cholesterol 56 mg
Sodium 120 mg
Carbohydrates 2 g
  Fiber 0 g
  Sugars 2 g
Protein 24 g
Dietary Exchanges
  3 lean meat

With the addition of a super-simple glaze, broiled steak becomes a special entrée. Gingered Bulgur and Dried Apricots (page 211) complements it well.

¼ **cup frozen orange juice concentrate**
½ **teaspoon ground coriander**
½ **teaspoon garlic powder**
⅛ **teaspoon pepper**
⅛ **teaspoon cayenne**
1 **1-pound boneless top sirloin steak, all visible fat discarded, cut into 4 pieces**
  Cooking spray
⅛ **teaspoon salt**

In a small bowl, stir together the orange juice concentrate, coriander, garlic powder, pepper, and cayenne. Pour about half the mixture into a separate small bowl.

Put the beef in a shallow glass dish. Brush the top side of the beef with all the orange juice mixture from one bowl. Cover the beef and refrigerate for 10 minutes. Set aside the remaining orange juice mixture.

About 20 minutes before serving time, preheat the broiler. Lightly spray the broiler pan and rack with cooking spray.

Transfer the beef to the rack.

Broil the beef with the seasoned side up about 4 inches from the heat for 8 minutes. Turn over. Using a clean basting brush, brush the top side with the remaining orange juice mixture. Broil for 8 to 10 minutes, or to the desired doneness.

Transfer the beef to a cutting board. Thinly slice on the diagonal. Sprinkle with the salt.

beef fajitas
IN LETTUCE WRAPS

SERVES 4
2 fajitas per serving

PREPARATION TIME
10 to 12 minutes

COOKING TIME
10 to 11 minutes

PER SERVING

Calories 185
Total Fat 3.5 g
  Saturated Fat 1.0 g
  Trans Fat 0.0 g
  Polyunsaturated Fat 0.5 g
  Monounsaturated Fat 2.0 g
Cholesterol 48 mg
Sodium 202 mg
Carbohydrates 14 g
  Fiber 3 g
  Sugars 7 g
Protein 23 g
Dietary Exchanges
  2 vegetable,
  ½ other carbohydrate,
  2½ lean meat

Add some crunch and cut the fat and sodium by wrapping these fajitas in lettuce leaves instead of the usual flour tortillas. Serve them with Chunky Salsa (page 32) and Homemade Corn Tortilla Chips (page 40).

    Cooking spray
12 ounces boneless top round steak, all visible fat discarded, thinly cut against the grain into strips 2 to 3 inches long
1 teaspoon canola or corn oil
1 large onion, thinly sliced
1 medium red, yellow, or green bell pepper, cut into strips
1 teaspoon bottled minced garlic or 2 medium garlic cloves, minced
2 tablespoons fresh lime juice
½ teaspoon ground cumin
¼ teaspoon salt
8 medium romaine or leaf lettuce leaves
½ cup fat-free sour cream

Lightly spray a large skillet with cooking spray. Heat over medium-high heat. Cook the beef for 2 to 3 minutes, or to the desired doneness, stirring frequently. Transfer to a plate. Wipe the skillet with paper towels if needed.

    Pour the oil into the skillet, swirling to coat the bottom. Cook the onion, bell pepper, and garlic, still over medium-high heat, for 3 minutes, or until the onion is soft, stirring frequently. Return the beef to the skillet.

    Stir in the lime juice, cumin, and salt. Cook for 3 minutes, or until heated through.

    Spoon the beef mixture onto the center of each lettuce leaf. Top with the sour cream. Fold the lettuce around the filling.

COOK'S TIP ON SLICING RAW MEAT
Slicing raw meat into thin strips will be easy if you put it in the freezer about 30 minutes before you plan to grab your favorite knife.

moroccan beef and barley

SERVES 4
2 cups per serving

PREPARATION TIME
10 minutes

COOKING TIME
1 hour 40 minutes

OR

SLOW-COOKER TIME
4 hours 30 minutes to
5 hours 30 minutes
on high *or* 8 hours
30 minutes to 10 hours
30 minutes on low

PER SERVING

Calories 303
Total Fat 3.0 g
  Saturated Fat 1.0 g
  Trans Fat 0.0 g
  Polyunsaturated Fat 0.5 g
  Monounsaturated Fat 1.0 g
Cholesterol 43 mg
Sodium 215 mg
Carbohydrates 44 g
  Fiber 9 g
  Sugars 12 g
Protein 26 g
Dietary Exchanges
  2 starch, 3 vegetable,
  2½ very lean meat

An unexpected combination of spices delightfully seasons this one-dish meal. Use your family's favorites for the frozen mixed vegetables.

Cooking spray
12 ounces boneless round steak, all visible fat discarded, cut into bite-size pieces
2 14.5-ounce cans no-salt-added diced tomatoes, undrained
1½ cups water
1 small onion, sliced and separated into rings
½ cup uncooked medium pearl barley
1 teaspoon sugar
1 teaspoon ground cumin
1 teaspoon ground ginger
1 teaspoon bottled minced garlic or 2 medium garlic cloves, minced
½ teaspoon ground turmeric
½ teaspoon paprika
½ teaspoon ground cinnamon
¼ teaspoon salt
10 ounces frozen mixed vegetables, any combination

Lightly spray a Dutch oven with cooking spray. Heat over medium-high heat. Cook the beef for 5 minutes, or until browned, stirring frequently.

Stir in the remaining ingredients except the mixed vegetables. Increase the heat to high and bring to a boil. Reduce the heat and simmer, covered, for 1 hour.

Stir in the mixed vegetables. Return to a simmer and simmer, covered, for 30 minutes, or until the beef, barley, and vegetables are tender and the liquid is absorbed. Stir before serving.

SLOW-COOKER METHOD

Put bite-size pieces of beef in a 3½- or 4-quart slow cooker without browning them. Add the remaining ingredients except the vegetables. Cook, covered, on high for 4 to 5 hours or on low for 8 to 10 hours, or until the beef is tender. Stir in the vegetables. Cook for 30 minutes, or until the vegetables are tender.

easy oven beef stew

SERVES 6
1 cup per serving

PREPARATION TIME
13 minutes

COOKING TIME
2 hours

OR

SLOW-COOKER TIME
4 hours 30 minutes to
5 hours 30 minutes on
high *or* 9 to 11 hours
on low

PER SERVING

Calories 266
Total Fat 3.0 g
  Saturated Fat 1.5 g
  Trans Fat 0.0 g
  Polyunsaturated Fat 0.5 g
  Monounsaturated Fat 1.5 g
Cholesterol 57 mg
Sodium 214 mg
Carbohydrates 28 g
  Fiber 3 g
  Sugars 5 g
Protein 30 g
Dietary Exchanges
  1½ starch, 2 vegetable,
  3 lean meat

Simply toss all the ingredients into a Dutch oven, put the stew in the oven, and forget about it for two hours, or let it cook all day in your slow cooker. No wonder we call it "easy"!

Cooking spray
¼ cup all-purpose flour
¼ teaspoon salt
¼ teaspoon pepper
1½ pounds boneless round steak, all visible fat discarded, cut into ½-inch cubes
3 cups water
2 medium potatoes, cut into bite-size pieces
9 ounces frozen whole baby carrots
8 ounces presliced button mushrooms (about 2½ cups)
1 cup frozen pearl onions
1 tablespoon plus 1 teaspoon very low sodium beef bouillon granules
1 teaspoon dried savory or thyme, crumbled
½ teaspoon garlic powder

Preheat the oven to 350°F. Lightly spray a Dutch oven with cooking spray.

In a large bowl, stir together the flour, salt, and pepper. Add the beef, turning to coat. Shake off any excess. Transfer to the Dutch oven.

Stir in the remaining ingredients.

Bake, covered, for 2 hours, or until the beef is tender, stirring once or twice.

SLOW-COOKER METHOD

Prepare the beef as directed above. Put the beef and remaining ingredients in a 3½- or 4-quart slow cooker. Cook, covered, on high for 4 hours 30 minutes to 5 hours 30 minutes or on low for 9 to 11 hours, or until the beef is tender.

quick-fix chicken-fried steak

SERVES 4
3 ounces beef and
2 tablespoons gravy
per serving

PREPARATION TIME
10 minutes

COOKING TIME
13 to 16 minutes

PER SERVING
Calories 236
Total Fat 5.0 g
  Saturated Fat 1.5 g
  Trans Fat 0.0 g
  Polyunsaturated Fat 0.5 g
  Monounsaturated Fat 3.0 g
Cholesterol 59 mg
Sodium 396 mg
Carbohydrates 16 g
  Fiber 1 g
  Sugars 3 g
Protein 30 g
Dietary Exchanges
  1 starch, 3 lean meat

Comfort food southern-style gets a healthy makeover in this version of a classic. The smoked paprika adds just enough difference to set this version apart without getting southerners up in arms!

  ½ cup low-fat buttermilk
  ½ cup all-purpose flour
  1 teaspoon smoked paprika
  ½ teaspoon garlic powder
  ½ teaspoon salt
  ½ teaspoon pepper
  4 cube steaks (about 4 ounces each), all visible fat discarded
  2 teaspoons olive oil
  ¾ cup fat-free milk

Pour the buttermilk into a medium shallow dish.

In a pie pan, stir together the flour, paprika, garlic powder, salt, and pepper. Measure out and set aside 1 tablespoon of the mixture.

Put the dish, pie pan, and a large plate in a row, assembly-line fashion. Dip 1 piece of beef in the buttermilk, turning to coat and letting any excess drip off. Dip in the flour mixture, turning to coat and gently shaking off any excess. Transfer to the plate. Repeat with the remaining pieces of beef.

In a large nonstick skillet, heat the oil over medium-high heat, swirling to coat the bottom. Cook the beef for 4 to 5 minutes on each side, or until browned on the outside and cooked through. Transfer to a separate large plate. Cover to keep warm.

Meanwhile, in a small bowl, whisk together the milk and reserved 1 tablespoon flour mixture (the mixture may be slightly lumpy). Pour into the skillet, scraping to dislodge any browned bits. Bring to a boil over medium-high heat, whisking constantly. Reduce the heat to medium low. Cook for 1 to 2 minutes, or until the gravy is thickened, whisking occasionally. Spoon over the beef.

espresso minute steaks

SERVES 4
3 ounces beef per serving

PREPARATION TIME
5 minutes

COOKING TIME
8 minutes

PER SERVING
Calories 158
Total Fat 5.0 g
  Saturated Fat 1.0 g
  Trans Fat 0.0 g
  Polyunsaturated Fat 1.0 g
  Monounsaturated Fat 2.5 g
Cholesterol 58 mg
Sodium 219 mg
Carbohydrates 1 g
  Fiber 0 g
  Sugars 1 g
Protein 26 g
Dietary Exchanges
  3 lean meat

Minute steaks, thin cuts of round steak, actually take about a minute and a half to cook. Talk about fast! A coffee-based reduction adds boldness to the dish.

½ cup strong coffee, or 1 teaspoon instant coffee granules dissolved in ½ cup water

2 teaspoons Worcestershire sauce (lowest sodium available)

2 teaspoons balsamic vinegar

¼ teaspoon salt

1 teaspoon canola or corn oil and 1 teaspoon canola or corn oil, divided use

4 minute steaks or thin round steaks (about 4 ounces each), all visible fat discarded

2 tablespoons finely chopped green onions (optional)

In a small bowl, stir together the coffee, Worcestershire sauce, vinegar, and salt. Set aside.

In a large nonstick skillet, heat 1 teaspoon oil over medium-high heat, swirling to coat the bottom. Cook 2 steaks for 1 minute. Turn over. Cook for 30 seconds, or until barely pink in the center. Transfer to a platter. Cover to keep warm. Repeat with the remaining 1 teaspoon oil and remaining steaks.

Stir the coffee mixture into the pan drippings, scraping to dislodge any browned bits. Bring to a boil over medium-high heat. Boil for 3 minutes, or until the mixture is reduced to 2 tablespoons, stirring frequently. Pour over the beef. Sprinkle with the green onions.

COOK'S TIP
Cooking the steaks in two batches ensures that they have more room and thus will brown, not stew.

cajun meat loaf

SERVES 6
1 slice per serving

PREPARATION TIME
10 minutes

COOKING TIME
45 minutes

OR

MICROWAVE TIME
8 to 10 minutes

STANDING TIME
5 minutes

PER SERVING

Calories 152
Total Fat 4.5 g
  Saturated Fat 1.5 g
  Trans Fat 0.0 g
  Polyunsaturated Fat 0.5 g
  Monounsaturated Fat 1.5 g
Cholesterol 42 mg
Sodium 298 mg
Carbohydrates 9 g
  Fiber 1 g
  Sugars 2 g
Protein 19 g
Dietary Exchanges
  ½ starch, 2½ lean meat

Spice up an everyday meat loaf with the rich flavors of the bayou. No-Chop Cajun Coleslaw (page 58) and corn are the perfect accompaniments. No loaf pan, no worries—this recipe calls for a baking pan, which also helps cut down on the cooking time!

Cooking spray
1 **pound extra-lean ground beef**
½ **cup chopped onion**
1 **medium rib of celery, chopped**
½ **medium red, yellow, or green bell pepper, chopped**
½ **cup plain dry bread crumbs
   (lowest sodium available)**
2 **large egg whites**
1 **tablespoon Worcestershire sauce
   (lowest sodium available)**
1 **teaspoon salt-free Cajun seasoning blend**
½ **teaspoon ground cumin**
¼ **teaspoon salt**
¼ **teaspoon pepper**
¼ **teaspoon cayenne**

Preheat the oven to 350°F. Lightly spray a 9-inch square baking pan with cooking spray.

In a large bowl, using your hands or a spoon, combine all the ingredients. Shape into a loaf about 8 × 5 inches. Transfer to the baking pan.

Bake for 45 minutes, or until the meat loaf registers 165°F on an instant-read thermometer and is no longer pink in the center. Remove from the oven. Let stand for 5 minutes before slicing.

MICROWAVE METHOD

Combine the ingredients as directed, but use a 9-inch glass pie pan instead of the baking pan. Shape the mixture into a 6-inch-wide ring with a 2-inch hole in the middle. Microwave, covered, on 100 percent power (high) for 8 to 10 minutes, or until the meat loaf registers 165°F on an instant-read thermometer and is no longer pink in the center. Let stand for 5 minutes before slicing.

healthy joes

WITH PASTA

SERVES 4

1¼ cups pasta and ½ cup "joe" mixture per serving

PREPARATION TIME
10 minutes

COOKING TIME
15 minutes

PER SERVING

Calories 401
Total Fat 7.0 g
  Saturated Fat 2.0 g
  Trans Fat 0.5 g
  Polyunsaturated Fat 1.0 g
  Monounsaturated Fat 2.5 g
Cholesterol 47 mg
Sodium 441 mg
Carbohydrates 59 g
  Fiber 10 g
  Sugars 9 g
Protein 29 g
Dietary Exchanges
  3 starch, 3 vegetable,
  2½ lean meat

As messy and delicious as traditional sloppy joes, our version is made with extra-lean beef and includes a shredded zucchini to add to your daily veggies.

8	ounces uncooked whole-grain spaghetti
12	ounces extra-lean ground beef
1	cup chopped onion
1	medium red, yellow, or green bell pepper, chopped
1½	cups meatless spaghetti sauce (lowest sodium available)
1	medium zucchini, shredded
1	tablespoon chili powder
1	teaspoon paprika
½	teaspoon bottled minced garlic or 1 medium garlic clove, minced
⅛	teaspoon salt

Prepare the pasta using the package directions, omitting the salt. Drain well in a colander. Transfer to a serving bowl and cover to keep warm. Set aside.

Meanwhile, in a large skillet, cook the beef, onion, and bell pepper over medium-high heat for 7 minutes, or until the beef is browned on the outside and no longer pink in the center, stirring occasionally to turn and break up the beef.

Stir in the remaining ingredients. Bring to a boil over high heat. Reduce the heat and simmer for 5 minutes. Spoon over the pasta.

southwest shepherd's pie

SERVES 8
heaping 1 cup
per serving

PREPARATION TIME
8 to 10 minutes

COOKING TIME
40 to 45 minutes

PER SERVING
Calories 218
Total Fat 2.5 g
  Saturated Fat 1.0 g
  Trans Fat 0.0 g
  Polyunsaturated Fat 0.0 g
  Monounsaturated Fat 0.5 g
Cholesterol 17 mg
Sodium 319 mg
Carbohydrates 36 g
  Fiber 4 g
  Sugars 8 g
Protein 15 g
Dietary Exchanges
  2½ starch, 1½ very lean
  meat

British shepherd's pie takes a trip to the Southwest, courtesy of kidney beans, corn, mild green chiles, and cumin. Add a salad to complement the meal.

8 ounces extra-lean ground beef
½ cup chopped onion
2 cups uncooked packaged instant mashed potatoes
2 cups water and ¼ cup water, divided use
¾ cup fat-free milk
1 15.5-ounce can no-salt-added kidney beans, rinsed and drained
1 12-ounce can no-salt-added whole-kernel corn, drained
1 10¾-ounce can low-fat condensed tomato soup (lowest sodium available)
1 4-ounce can chopped green chiles, drained
1 teaspoon ground cumin
⅛ teaspoon salt
⅛ teaspoon pepper
¼ cup shredded fat-free Cheddar cheese

Preheat the oven to 375°F.

In a large skillet, cook the beef and onion over medium-high heat for 5 minutes, or until the beef is browned on the outside and the onion is soft, stirring occasionally to turn and break up the beef.

Meanwhile, prepare the potatoes using the package directions, using 2 cups water and ¾ cup milk and omitting any margarine and salt.

Stir the beans, corn, soup, chiles, cumin, salt, pepper, and remaining ¼ cup water into the beef mixture. Cook for 7 minutes, or until heated through, stirring occasionally. Transfer to a 2-quart casserole dish.

Drop the potato mixture in mounds or spread it over the beef mixture.

Bake for 25 to 30 minutes, or until hot. Sprinkle with the Cheddar.

pork roast

WITH HORSERADISH AND HERBS

SERVES 8
3 ounces pork
per serving

PREPARATION TIME
5 minutes

COOKING TIME
1 hour

STANDING TIME
3 minutes

PER SERVING

Calories 135
Total Fat 5.5 g
  Saturated Fat 2.0 g
  Trans Fat 0.0 g
  Polyunsaturated Fat 0.5 g
  Monounsaturated Fat 2.5 g
Cholesterol 49 mg
Sodium 187 mg
Carbohydrates 0 g
  Fiber 0 g
  Sugars 0 g
Protein 19 g
Dietary Exchanges
  3 lean meat

Dress up this entrée with a sophisticated side, such as Strawberry-Spinach Salad with Champagne Dressing (page 56), or dress it down with a homey side, such as German-Style Noodles (page 216).

    Cooking spray
1 2-pound boneless pork rib roast or loin roast, all visible fat discarded
1 teaspoon bottled white horseradish, drained
½ teaspoon dried marjoram, crumbled
½ teaspoon dried basil, crumbled
½ teaspoon dried oregano, crumbled
¼ teaspoon salt

Preheat the oven to 350°F.

Put the pork in a medium shallow baking pan. Spread the horseradish over the top of the pork.

In a small bowl, stir together the marjoram, basil, oregano, and salt. Sprinkle over the horseradish.

Roast for 1 hour, or until the pork registers 145°F on an instant-read thermometer. Remove from the oven and let stand for 3 minutes, or until the desired doneness.

pork and rhubarb bake

SERVES 4
⅔ cup per serving

PREPARATION TIME
10 minutes

COOKING TIME
28 to 33 minutes

PER SERVING
Calories 207
Total Fat 5.5 g
 Saturated Fat 2.0 g
 Trans Fat 0.0 g
 Polyunsaturated Fat 0.5 g
 Monounsaturated Fat 2.5 g
Cholesterol 49 mg
Sodium 184 mg
Carbohydrates 20 g
 Fiber 2 g
 Sugars 14 g
Protein 20 g
Dietary Exchanges
 2½ other carbohydrate,
 2½ lean meat

Browned pork cubes are sandwiched between layers of rhubarb in this unusual dish. Serve it with sides of brown rice and green beans.

Cooking spray
12 **ounces boneless pork loin roast or chops, all visible fat discarded, cut into bite-size pieces**
1 **to 1½ pounds rhubarb, cut into bite-size pieces (about 3 cups), or 16 ounces frozen unsweetened cut rhubarb, thawed and drained if frozen**
¼ **cup sugar**
2 **tablespoons all-purpose flour**
½ **teaspoon ground cinnamon**
¼ **teaspoon salt**

Preheat the oven to 350°F. Lightly spray a large skillet with cooking spray.

Heat the skillet over medium-high heat. Cook the pork for 5 minutes, or until browned, stirring frequently.

In a large bowl, stir together the remaining ingredients. Spoon half the rhubarb mixture into a 1½-quart casserole dish. Spoon the pork over the rhubarb mixture. Top with the remaining rhubarb mixture.

Bake, covered, for 20 to 25 minutes, or until the pork is the desired doneness and the rhubarb is tender.

hearty pork and onion stew

SERVES 6
1¼ cups per serving

PREPARATION TIME
13 to 15 minutes

COOKING TIME
1 hour 30 minutes

OR

SLOW-COOKER TIME
4 to 5 hours on high *or*
8 to 10 hours on low

PER SERVING
Calories 285
Total Fat 7.5 g
  Saturated Fat 2.5 g
  Trans Fat 0.0 g
  Polyunsaturated Fat 0.5 g
  Monounsaturated Fat 3.0 g
Cholesterol 65 mg
Sodium 201 mg
Carbohydrates 22 g
  Fiber 2 g
  Sugars 5 g
Protein 29 g
Dietary Exchanges
  ½ starch, 2 vegetable,
  3 lean meat

Whether you bake or slow-cook this stew, you can be confident that your family will enjoy it.

    Cooking spray
⅓ cup all-purpose flour
¼ teaspoon salt
⅛ teaspoon pepper
1½ pounds boneless pork loin roast, all visible fat discarded, cut into ½-inch cubes
16 ounces frozen pearl onions
1 12-ounce can light beer or nonalcoholic beer
1¼ cups fat-free, low-sodium chicken broth
10 ounces frozen chopped spinach, slightly thawed, broken into chunks
2 tablespoons red wine vinegar
1 tablespoon firmly packed brown sugar
1 teaspoon caraway seeds
1 teaspoon bottled minced garlic or 2 medium garlic cloves, minced
1 medium dried bay leaf

Preheat the oven to 350°F. Lightly spray a Dutch oven or a 3-quart glass casserole dish with cooking spray.

In a large bowl, stir together the flour, salt, and pepper. Add half the pork, turning to coat and gently shaking off any excess. Transfer the pork to the Dutch oven. Repeat with the remaining pork.

Stir in the remaining ingredients.

Bake, covered, for 1 hour 30 minutes, or until the pork is tender and the desired doneness, stirring occasionally. Discard the bay leaf before serving the stew.

SLOW-COOKER METHOD

Prepare the pork as directed above. Put the pork and remaining ingredients in a 3½- or 4-quart slow cooker. Cook, covered, on high for 4 to 5 hours or on low for 8 to 10 hours, or until the pork is tender and the desired doneness. Discard the bay leaf before serving the stew.

three-pepper pork

SERVES 4
3 ounces pork
per serving

PREPARATION TIME
10 to 13 minutes

COOKING TIME
12 minutes

PER SERVING
Calories 219
Total Fat 8.5 g
    Saturated Fat 3.0 g
    Trans Fat 0.0 g
    Polyunsaturated Fat 1.5 g
    Monounsaturated Fat 3.5 g
Cholesterol 65 mg
Sodium 148 mg
Carbohydrates 9 g
    Fiber 2 g
    Sugars 5 g
Protein 26 g
Dietary Exchanges
    2 vegetable, 3 lean meat

This recipe may sound spicy, but it isn't—unless you want to ramp up the heat (see Cook's Tip below). The triple-pepper flavor comes from red bell pepper, yellow bell pepper, and mild poblano pepper. Asian flair is added with a mixture of soy sauce, fresh ginger, sesame oil, and rice wine vinegar.

Cooking spray
1   **pound boneless pork loin roast or chops, all visible fat discarded, cut into strips**
1   **medium red bell pepper, cut into strips**
1   **medium yellow bell pepper, cut into strips**
1   **medium poblano pepper, chopped**
1   **tablespoon sugar**
1   **tablespoon soy sauce (lowest sodium available)**
1   **teaspoon peeled grated gingerroot**
1   **teaspoon toasted sesame oil**
1   **teaspoon plain rice wine vinegar**

Lightly spray a large skillet with cooking spray. Heat over medium-high heat. Cook the pork for 5 minutes, or until slightly pink in the center, stirring occasionally.

Stir in all the peppers. Cook for 3 minutes, or until the peppers are tender-crisp, stirring occasionally.

In a small bowl, stir together the remaining ingredients. Stir into the pork mixture. Cook for 2 minutes, or until heated through, stirring constantly.

COOK'S TIP
If you like fiery food, you may want to spice up this recipe by replacing the poblano with hot chile peppers, such as jalapeño or serrano, to taste.

sesame pork tenderloin

SERVES 6
3 ounces pork
per serving

PREPARATION TIME
7 minutes

COOKING TIME
40 to 45 minutes

STANDING TIME
3 minutes

PER SERVING
Calories 147
Total Fat 3.5 g
    Saturated Fat 1.0 g
    Trans Fat 0.0 g
    Polyunsaturated Fat 1.0 g
    Monounsaturated Fat 1.5 g
Cholesterol 74 mg
Sodium 128 mg
Carbohydrates 3 g
    Fiber 0 g
    Sugars 3 g
Protein 24 g
Dietary Exchanges
    3 lean meat

For a festive Asian meal, pair this so-easy pork tenderloin with Spinach and Brown Rice Soup with Ginger (page 46) and stir-fried vegetables garnished with curls of lemon zest.

    Cooking spray
1½ pounds pork tenderloin, all visible fat discarded
  1 tablespoon light molasses
  1 tablespoon soy sauce (lowest sodium available)
 ¼ teaspoon toasted sesame oil
  1 tablespoon sesame seeds

Preheat the oven to 425°F. Lightly spray a large shallow baking pan with cooking spray.

Put the pork in the baking pan.

In a small bowl, stir together the molasses, soy sauce, and sesame oil. Brush all over the pork. Sprinkle the pork with the sesame seeds.

Roast for 40 to 45 minutes, or until the pork registers 145°F on an instant-read thermometer. Remove from the oven and let stand for 3 minutes, or until the desired doneness. Cut crosswise into slices.

COOK'S TIP
If your tenderloin comes in two pieces, use wooden toothpicks to secure them together.

pesto pork pinwheels

SERVES 4
3 ounces pork
per serving

PREPARATION TIME
8 to 10 minutes

COOKING TIME
30 to 35 minutes

STANDING TIME
3 minutes

PER SERVING
Calories 136
Total Fat 3.5 g
  Saturated Fat 1.0 g
  Trans Fat 0.0 g
  Polyunsaturated Fat 0.5 g
  Monounsaturated Fat 1.5 g
Cholesterol 74 mg
Sodium 75 mg
Carbohydrates 0 g
  Fiber 0 g
  Sugars 0 g
Protein 24 g
Dietary Exchanges
  3 lean meat

When you try this dish, you'll be pleasantly surprised at how good a two-ingredient recipe can be. Serve it with Fresh Herb Polenta (page 221) and zucchini.

1 **1-pound pork tenderloin, all visible fat discarded, butterflied and flattened to ¼-inch thickness**
1 **tablespoon Crunchy Basil-Parmesan Pesto (page 103) or commercial pesto (lowest sodium available)**

Preheat the oven to 425°F.

Lay the pork flat. Spread the pesto over the pork. Roll up from one of the short ends and tie with string in several places to secure. Transfer to a medium shallow baking pan.

Roast for 30 to 35 minutes, or until the pork registers 145°F on an instant-read thermometer. Remove from the oven and let stand for 3 minutes, or until the desired doneness. Cut crosswise into slices.

pork medallions
WITH SAUTÉED MUSHROOMS

SERVES 4
3 medallions and
2 tablespoons mushroom
mixture per serving

PREPARATION TIME
10 minutes

COOKING TIME
16 to 17 minutes

PER SERVING
Calories 151
Total Fat 4.0 g
    Saturated Fat 1.0 g
    Trans Fat 0.0 g
    Polyunsaturated Fat 1.0 g
    Monounsaturated Fat 1.5 g
Cholesterol 74 mg
Sodium 233 mg
Carbohydrates 3 g
    Fiber 1 g
    Sugars 2 g
Protein 26 g
Dietary Exchanges
    3 lean meat

*Although the sherry is optional, use it if possible—it adds a
very pleasant flavor and complements the rosemary.*

Cooking spray

1   **1-pound pork tenderloin, all visible fat discarded,
    cut into 12 slices and flattened to ¾-inch
    thickness**

8   **ounces presliced button mushrooms
    (about 2½ cups)**

2   **medium green onions, sliced**

1   **tablespoon light tub margarine**

1   **teaspoon finely snipped fresh rosemary or
    ¼ teaspoon dried, crushed**

¼   **teaspoon salt**

1   **tablespoon dry sherry (optional)**

Lightly spray a large skillet with cooking spray. Heat
over medium-high heat. Cook half the pork for
3 minutes on each side, or until it registers 145°F on
an instant-read thermometer. Transfer to a large plate.
Cover to keep warm. Repeat with the remaining pork.

   In the same skillet, cook the remaining ingredients
except the sherry over medium heat for 2 to 3 minutes,
or until the mushrooms are soft, stirring occasionally.
Stir in the sherry. Spoon over the pork.

maple-bourbon pork medallions

SERVES 4
3 medallions and
2 tablespoons sauce
per serving

PREPARATION TIME
7 minutes

COOKING TIME
18 to 20 minutes

PER SERVING
Calories 256
Total Fat 3.0 g
    Saturated Fat 1.0 g
    Trans Fat 0.0 g
    Polyunsaturated Fat 0.5 g
    Monounsaturated Fat 1.0 g
Cholesterol 74 mg
Sodium 218 mg
Carbohydrates 21 g
    Fiber 0 g
    Sugars 19 g
Protein 24 g
Dietary Exchanges
    1½ other carbohydrate,
    3 very lean meat

You won't want to waste a drop of this special sauce, so serve your favorite whole-grain pasta on the side and drizzle the extra sauce over it.

⅓ cup maple syrup

⅓ cup bourbon or unsweetened apple juice

2 tablespoons whole-grain or Dijon mustard (lowest sodium available)

2 tablespoons no-salt-added ketchup
Cooking spray

1 1-pound pork tenderloin, all visible fat discarded, cut into 12 slices and flattened to ¾-inch thickness

In a small bowl, stir together the maple syrup, bourbon, mustard, and ketchup. Set aside.

Lightly spray a large skillet with cooking spray. Heat over medium-high heat. Cook half the pork for 3 minutes on each side, or until it registers 145°F on an instant-read thermometer. Transfer to a plate. Cover to keep warm. Repeat with the remaining pork.

In the same skillet, cook the syrup mixture, still over medium-high heat, for 4 minutes, or until bubbly, stirring frequently. Cook for 1 to 2 minutes, or until thickened to the desired consistency, stirring constantly. Spoon over the pork.

pork chops

WITH HONEY-LEMON SAUCE

SERVES 4
3 ounces pork and
2 tablespoons sauce
per serving

PREPARATION TIME
5 minutes

COOKING TIME
20 minutes

PER SERVING
Calories 255
Total Fat 8.0 g
   Saturated Fat 3.0 g
   Trans Fat 0.0 g
   Polyunsaturated Fat 1.0 g
   Monounsaturated Fat 3.5 g
Cholesterol 72 mg
Sodium 263 mg
Carbohydrates 19 g
   Fiber 0 g
   Sugars 18 g
Protein 26 g
Dietary Exchanges
   1½ other carbohydrate,
   3 lean meat

Too tasty to limit to just this one dish, this honey-lemon sauce is excellent over chicken or turkey, too.

   Cooking spray
 4 **boneless pork loin chops (about 4 ounces each), ½ to ¾ inch thick, all visible fat discarded, halved**

SAUCE
 ¼ **cup honey**
 ¼ **cup fresh lemon juice**
 2 **tablespoons soy sauce (lowest sodium available)**
 ½ **teaspoon bottled minced garlic or 1 medium garlic clove, minced**

Lightly spray a large skillet with cooking spray. Heat over medium-high heat. Cook the pork for 1 minute on each side. Reduce the heat to medium. Cook for 8 minutes. Turn over. Cook for 5 minutes, or until the pork registers 145°F on an instant-read thermometer. Transfer to a large plate. Cover to keep warm.

   Meanwhile, in a small bowl, stir together the sauce ingredients. Set aside.

   When the pork is done, pour the sauce into the same skillet. Cook over medium-high heat for 3 minutes, or until thickened to the desired consistency, stirring occasionally. Spoon over the pork.

tropical pork chops

SERVES 4

3 ounces pork
per serving

PREPARATION TIME
8 minutes

MARINATING TIME
24 hours

COOKING TIME
7 to 9 minutes

STANDING TIME
3 minutes

PER SERVING

Calories 156
Total Fat 7.0 g
 Saturated Fat 2.5 g
 Trans Fat 0.0 g
 Polyunsaturated Fat 0.5 g
 Monounsaturated Fat 3.5 g
Cholesterol 58 mg
Sodium 199 mg
Carbohydrates 0 g
 Fiber 0 g
 Sugars 0 g
Protein 21 g
Dietary Exchanges
 3 lean meat

Ginger, cloves, and nutmeg—plus some crushed red pepper flakes for a dash of heat—flavor the pineapple juice marinade in this dish. Note that the pork chops need to marinate for about a day.

MARINADE

½ cup fat-free, low-sodium chicken broth
½ cup pineapple juice
2 tablespoons firmly packed light brown sugar
2 tablespoons fresh lime juice
½ teaspoon ground ginger
¼ teaspoon ground cloves
¼ teaspoon salt
¼ teaspoon bottled minced garlic or ½ medium garlic clove, minced
⅛ teaspoon ground nutmeg
⅛ teaspoon crushed red pepper flakes

4 boneless pork loin chops (about 4 ounces each), about ¾ inch thick, all visible fat discarded
Cooking spray

In a large shallow glass dish, stir together the marinade ingredients. Add the pork, turning to coat. Cover and refrigerate for about 24 hours, turning occasionally.

About 20 minutes before serving time, lightly spray a broiler pan and rack with cooking spray. Preheat the broiler.

Drain the pork, discarding the marinade.

Broil the pork about 4 inches from the heat for 4 minutes. Turn over and broil for 3 to 5 minutes, or until it registers 145°F on an instant-read thermometer. Remove from the broiler. Let stand for 3 minutes, or until the desired doneness.

pork chop and sweet potato skillet

SERVES 4
3 ounces pork and heaping ¾ cup vegetables per serving

PREPARATION TIME
10 minutes

COOKING TIME
40 minutes

STANDING TIME
3 minutes

PER SERVING
Calories 260
Total Fat 6.5 g
  Saturated Fat 2.5 g
  Trans Fat 0.0 g
  Polyunsaturated Fat 0.5 g
  Monounsaturated Fat 3.0 g
Cholesterol 67 mg
Sodium 254 mg
Carbohydrates 23 g
  Fiber 4 g
  Sugars 10 g
Protein 26 g
Dietary Exchanges
  1 starch, 2 vegetable,
  3 lean meat

The acidity of the tomatoes and the sweetness of the potato make just the right balance of flavors for this dish.

Cooking spray
4 boneless pork loin chops (about 4 ounces each), ½ to ¾ inch thick, all visible fat discarded
1 large sweet potato, chopped
1 medium onion, chopped
1 15.5-ounce can no-salt-added stewed tomatoes, undrained
½ teaspoon dried basil, crumbled
½ teaspoon dried oregano, crumbled
½ teaspoon bottled minced garlic or 1 medium garlic clove, minced
¼ teaspoon salt

Lightly spray a large skillet with cooking spray. Heat over medium-high heat. Cook the pork for 5 minutes on each side, or until browned. Remove from the skillet.

Put the sweet potato and onion in the skillet. Place the pork on top. Pour in the tomatoes with liquid. Sprinkle with the basil, oregano, garlic, and salt. Increase the heat to high and bring to a boil. Reduce the heat and simmer, covered, for 25 minutes, or until the sweet potato is tender and the pork registers 145°F on an instant-read thermometer. Remove from the heat. Let stand, uncovered, for 3 minutes.

double-apricot and ham kebabs

SERVES 4
2 kebabs per serving

PREPARATION TIME
15 minutes

COOKING TIME
15 minutes

OR

MICROWAVE TIME
5 to 6 minutes

PER SERVING
Calories 195
Total Fat 2.0 g
  Saturated Fat 0.5 g
  Trans Fat 0.0 g
  Polyunsaturated Fat 0.0 g
  Monounsaturated Fat 1.0 g
Cholesterol 24 mg
Sodium 480 mg
Carbohydrates 34 g
  Fiber 2 g
  Sugars 28 g
Protein 10 g
Dietary Exchanges
  2 fruit, 1½ very lean meat

This version of dinner-on-a-stick features ham, fruit, and red bell pepper glazed with an apricot mixture.

¼ **cup all-fruit apricot spread**

1 **tablespoon white wine vinegar or cider vinegar**

¼ **teaspoon dry mustard**

8 **ounces lower-sodium, low-fat ham, all visible fat discarded, cut into 16 bite-size cubes**

16 **pineapple chunks from one 20-ounce can pineapple chunks in their own juice, drained**

16 **dried apricot halves**

1 **medium red bell pepper, cut into 16 squares**

Soak eight 10-inch wooden skewers in cold water for at least 10 minutes to keep them from charring, or use metal skewers.

Preheat the oven to 400°F.

In a small saucepan, stir together the apricot spread, vinegar, and mustard. Cook over low heat while preparing the kebabs, stirring occasionally.

On each skewer, thread 1 ham chunk, 1 pineapple chunk, 1 apricot half, and 1 bell pepper piece. Repeat. Transfer to a shallow glass baking dish large enough to hold the kebabs in a single layer. Brush the kebabs with the apricot mixture, reserving any remaining.

Bake the kebabs for 15 minutes, brushing occasionally with any remaining apricot mixture.

MICROWAVE METHOD

Prepare the recipe as directed, but use eight 10-inch wooden skewers or other microwaveable skewers. In a 1-cup microwaveable bowl, microwave the apricot mixture on 100 percent power (high) for 30 to 60 seconds, or until hot. Arrange the kebabs on a 9-inch glass pie pan or other microwaveable plate. Brush the kebabs with the apricot mixture. Microwave on high for 2 minutes. Brush with any remaining apricot mixture. Microwave on high for 2 to 3 minutes, or until heated through.

rosemary lamb chops

WITH LEMON SAUCE

SERVES 4
3 ounces lamb and
1½ tablespoons sauce
per serving

PREPARATION TIME
10 minutes

COOKING TIME
8 to 11 minutes

PER SERVING
Calories 152
Total Fat 6.5 g
  Saturated Fat 2.5 g
  Trans Fat 0.0 g
  Polyunsaturated Fat 0.5 g
  Monounsaturated Fat 3.0 g
Cholesterol 64 mg
Sodium 233 mg
Carbohydrates 1 g
  Fiber 0 g
  Sugars 0 g
Protein 20 g
Dietary Exchanges
  3 lean meat

Rub tiny bits of rosemary into lamb chops to impart wonderful flavor, then top the broiled lamb with a thick, lemony sauce. Serve the lamb with Savory Sweet Potato Sauté (page 228) and a crunchy green salad.

Cooking spray

1 tablespoon finely snipped fresh rosemary or 1 teaspoon dried, crushed

4 boneless lamb leg sirloin chops (about 4 ounces each), about ¾ inch thick, all visible fat discarded

⅓ cup fat-free, low-sodium chicken broth

1 teaspoon cornstarch

¼ teaspoon grated lemon zest

1 tablespoon fresh lemon juice

1 teaspoon Dijon mustard (lowest sodium available)

¼ teaspoon salt

Preheat the broiler. Lightly spray the broiler pan and rack with cooking spray.

Sprinkle the rosemary over both sides of the lamb. Using your fingertips, gently press the rosemary so it adheres to the lamb.

Broil the lamb about 4 inches from the heat for 5 to 6 minutes. Turn over. Broil for 3 to 5 minutes, or to the desired doneness.

Meanwhile, in a small saucepan, whisk together the broth and cornstarch. Whisk in the lemon zest, lemon juice, mustard, and salt. Cook over medium heat for 5 minutes, or until thickened to the desired consistency, whisking constantly. Serve over the lamb.

curried lamb stroganoff

SERVES 4
¾ cup stroganoff and
⅓ cup rice per serving

PREPARATION TIME
10 minutes

COOKING TIME
18 minutes

PER SERVING
Calories 289
Total Fat 5.5 g
  Saturated Fat 1.5 g
  Trans Fat 0.0 g
  Polyunsaturated Fat 1.0 g
  Monounsaturated Fat 2.0 g
Cholesterol 58 mg
Sodium 236 mg
Carbohydrates 38 g
  Fiber 3 g
  Sugars 12 g
Protein 22 g
Dietary Exchanges
  1½ starch, 1 fruit,
  2½ lean meat

This well-seasoned stroganoff is served with a raisin-studded brown rice mixture that cooks while you prepare the rest of the meal.

1   cup uncooked instant brown rice
¼   cup raisins or dried currants
12   ounces lean ground lamb
1   medium Granny Smith or other tart apple, peeled and chopped
1   small onion, chopped
¾   cup fat-free, low-sodium chicken broth
1   tablespoon plus 1 to 2 teaspoons curry powder
1   teaspoon bottled minced garlic or 2 medium garlic cloves, minced
¼   teaspoon salt
¼   teaspoon ground cinnamon
⅛   teaspoon pepper
¼   cup fat-free sour cream or fat-free plain yogurt
1   tablespoon all-purpose flour

Prepare the rice using the package directions, omitting the salt and margarine and adding the raisins.

Meanwhile, in a large skillet, cook the lamb over medium-high heat for 7 minutes, or until brown, stirring occasionally to turn and break up the lamb. Drain well. Return to the skillet.

Stir the apple, onion, broth, curry powder, garlic, salt, cinnamon, and pepper into the lamb. Increase the heat to high and bring to a boil. Reduce the heat and simmer, covered, for 5 minutes.

In a small bowl, whisk together the sour cream and flour. Stir into the lamb mixture. Cook over low heat for 3 minutes, or until the desired consistency, stirring constantly. Serve over the rice mixture.

kiwi veal

SERVES 4
3 ounces veal and
2 tablespoons sauce
per serving

PREPARATION TIME
5 minutes

COOKING TIME
5 minutes

PER SERVING
Calories 232
Total Fat 2.0 g
 Saturated Fat 0.5 g
 Trans Fat 0.0 g
 Polyunsaturated Fat 0.5 g
 Monounsaturated Fat 0.5 g
Cholesterol 89 mg
Sodium 218 mg
Carbohydrates 29 g
 Fiber 1 g
 Sugars 22 g
Protein 24 g
Dietary Exchanges
 2 other carbohydrate,
 3 very lean meat

Tomato preserves are not as sweet as other preserves and are the perfect balance to the kiwifruit in this recipe. The twosome makes a fabulous yet simple sauce for veal.

½ cup tomato preserves
1 medium kiwifruit, peeled and chopped
¼ teaspoon salt
   Cooking spray
1 pound veal scaloppine, cut about ¼ inch thick

In a small saucepan, stir together the tomato preserves, kiwifruit, and salt. Cook over low heat for 3 minutes, or until heated through, stirring occasionally.

Meanwhile, lightly spray a large skillet with cooking spray. Heat over medium-high heat. Cook the veal for 2 minutes on each side, or until tender. Serve topped with the sauce.

COOK'S TIP
Tomato preserves are made with tomatoes, corn syrup, and lemon juice. Look for tomato preserves with other preserves at the supermarket. If they're not available, choose another lower-sugar preserve, such as apricot or jalapeño.

veal scaloppine
IN SHIITAKE CREAM SAUCE

SERVES 4
3 ounces veal and
⅓ cup sauce
per serving

PREPARATION TIME
10 minutes

COOKING TIME
19 minutes

PER SERVING
Calories 226
Total Fat 2.5 g
  Saturated Fat 1.0 g
  Trans Fat 0.0 g
  Polyunsaturated Fat 0.5 g
  Monounsaturated Fat 0.5 g
Cholesterol 92 mg
Sodium 335 mg
Carbohydrates 17 g
  Fiber 2 g
  Sugars 13 g
Protein 33 g
Dietary Exchanges
  1 fat-free milk, 1 vegetable,
  3 very lean meat

This elegant entrée is worthy of a special-occasion dinner or celebration. Try it with Sugar-Kissed Snow Peas and Carrots (page 220) and whole-wheat orzo.

Cooking spray
1 pound veal scaloppine, cut about ¼ inch thick
8 ounces shiitake mushrooms, stems discarded, sliced, or presliced button mushrooms
4 medium green onions, sliced
1 teaspoon bottled minced garlic or 2 medium garlic cloves, minced
2 teaspoons all-purpose flour
½ teaspoon chopped fresh thyme or ¼ teaspoon dried, crumbled
¼ teaspoon salt
⅛ teaspoon pepper
1 12-ounce can fat-free evaporated milk
1 tablespoon dry sherry (optional)

Lightly spray a large skillet with cooking spray. Heat over medium-high heat. Cook the veal for 2 minutes on each side, or until tender. Transfer to a large plate. Cover to keep warm.

Lightly spray the same skillet with cooking spray. Cook the mushrooms, green onions, and garlic over medium heat for 5 minutes, or until the mushrooms are soft, stirring occasionally.

Stir in the flour, thyme, salt, and pepper. Pour in the evaporated milk all at once, stirring to combine. Cook for 4 minutes, or until the desired consistency, stirring constantly. Stir in the sherry.

Return the veal to the skillet, turning to coat. Cook for 3 minutes, or until heated through.

COOK'S TIP
You can make the sauce for this dish ahead of time and refrigerate it. To serve, reheat the sauce in a skillet over low heat while cooking the veal.

vegetarian entrées

spicy penne
WITH GREENS AND BEANS

SERVES 6
1½ cups per serving

PREPARATION TIME
8 to 9 minutes

COOKING TIME
23 to 26 minutes

PER SERVING
Calories 326
Total Fat 2.5 g
  Saturated Fat 0.0 g
  Trans Fat 0.0 g
  Polyunsaturated Fat 0.5 g
  Monounsaturated Fat 1.5 g
Cholesterol 0 mg
Sodium 257 mg
Carbohydrates 62 g
  Fiber 13 g
  Sugars 12 g
Protein 15 g
Dietary Exchanges
  3½ starch, 2 vegetable,
  1 very lean meat

This hearty mixture of whole-grain penne, collard greens, and black beans will really hit the spot! Adding the collard greens to the pot of water before it is brought to a boil saves time.

3 quarts water and ½ cup water, divided use
8 ounces collard greens, any large stems discarded, chopped (about 5 cups)
8 ounces dried whole-grain penne (about 3 cups)
2 teaspoons olive oil
½ cup chopped onion
1 medium carrot, sliced
1 teaspoon finely snipped fresh rosemary
1 teaspoon snipped fresh thyme
½ teaspoon crushed red pepper flakes
2 15.5-ounce cans no-salt-added black beans, rinsed and drained
2 cups no-salt-added crushed tomatoes, undrained
¼ cup balsamic vinegar
½ teaspoon salt
   Red hot-pepper sauce to taste (optional)

In a soup pot, bring 3 quarts water and the collard greens to a boil, covered, over high heat. Stir in the pasta. Cook, uncovered, using the package directions and omitting the salt. Drain well in a colander.

Meanwhile, in a large skillet, heat the oil over medium-high heat, swirling to coat the bottom. Cook the onion, carrot, rosemary, thyme, and red pepper flakes for 3 to 4 minutes, or until the onion is soft, stirring frequently.

Stir in the beans, tomatoes with liquid, vinegar, salt, and remaining ½ cup water. Reduce the heat to medium low. Cook for 3 minutes, or until heated through, stirring frequently. Remove from the heat.

Stir in the pasta mixture. Serve with the hot-pepper sauce.

rotini
WITH CREAMY BASIL-EDAMAME SAUCE

SERVES 4
1½ cups per serving

PREPARATION TIME
12 minutes

COOKING TIME
9 to 11 minutes

PER SERVING
Calories 316
Total Fat 6.5 g
  Saturated Fat 0.5 g
  Trans Fat 0.0 g
  Polyunsaturated Fat 1.0 g
  Monounsaturated Fat 2.5 g
Cholesterol 4 mg
Sodium 243 mg
Carbohydrates 51 g
  Fiber 9 g
  Sugars 7 g
Protein 17 g
Dietary Exchanges
  3 starch, 1 vegetable,
  1 lean meat

Edamame is the surprise ingredient in the thick and wonderful sauce that coats whole-grain pasta in this dish.

- 8 **ounces dried whole-grain rotini or rotelle pasta (about 3 cups)**
- 6 **ounces frozen shelled edamame (green soybeans), thawed**
- ½ **cup loosely packed fresh basil (about ¾ ounce)**
- ¼ **cup low-fat ricotta cheese**
- 1 **tablespoon fresh lemon juice**
- 1 **teaspoon bottled minced garlic or 2 medium garlic cloves, minced**
- 1 **teaspoon olive oil and 1 teaspoon olive oil, divided use**
- ¼ **teaspoon salt**
- 1 **tablespoon water (if needed)**
- 8 **ounces sliced baby bella mushrooms (about 2½ cups)**
- 1 **cup chopped onion**
- 2 **tablespoons crumbled fat-free feta cheese**

Prepare the pasta using the package directions, omitting the salt. Drain well in a colander.

Meanwhile, in a food processor or blender, process the edamame, basil, ricotta, lemon juice, garlic, 1 teaspoon oil, and the salt for 40 seconds, or until smooth, scraping the side of the bowl once. If the mixture is too thick, add the water and process until blended. Set aside.

In a medium nonstick skillet, heat the remaining 1 teaspoon oil over medium-high heat, swirling to coat the bottom. Cook the mushrooms and onion for 3 minutes, or until soft, stirring frequently. Transfer to a large bowl.

Add the pasta and the edamame mixture to the mushroom mixture, stirring gently to coat. Serve sprinkled with the feta.

tangy yogurt-tomato fusilli

SERVES 4
1½ cups per serving

PREPARATION TIME
8 minutes

COOKING TIME
13 to 15 minutes

PER SERVING

Calories 302
Total Fat 3.5 g
  Saturated Fat 0.0 g
  Trans Fat 0.0 g
  Polyunsaturated Fat 0.5 g
  Monounsaturated Fat 0.5 g
Cholesterol 0 mg
Sodium 218 mg
Carbohydrates 52 g
  Fiber 9 g
  Sugars 8 g
Protein 17 g
Dietary Exchanges
  3 starch, 1 vegetable,
  1 very lean meat

Edamame add a delightfully chewy texture and bright color to this whole-grain pasta dish.

8 ounces dried whole-grain fusilli (about 3½ cups)
1 14.5-ounce can no-salt-added diced tomatoes, undrained
1 teaspoon bottled minced garlic or 2 medium garlic cloves, minced
1 teaspoon dried rosemary, crushed
1 cup frozen shelled edamame (green soybeans)
2 teaspoons capers, drained and chopped
½ teaspoon grated lemon zest
¼ teaspoon salt
¼ teaspoon pepper
6 ounces fat-free plain Greek yogurt

Prepare the pasta using the package directions, omitting the salt. Drain well in a colander. Transfer to a large bowl.

Meanwhile, in a large nonstick skillet, cook the tomatoes with liquid, garlic, and rosemary over medium-high heat for 5 minutes, stirring occasionally.

Stir in the remaining ingredients except the yogurt. Bring to a simmer, still over medium-high heat. Reduce the heat and simmer for 5 to 6 minutes, or until most of the liquid has evaporated, stirring occasionally. Remove from the heat.

Stir the yogurt into the edamame mixture. Stir into the pasta. Serve immediately to keep the pasta from absorbing the sauce.

mediterranean penne

WITH PINE NUT TOMATO SAUCE AND FETA

SERVES 4
1½ cups per serving

PREPARATION TIME
11 to 13 minutes

COOKING TIME
23 to 26 minutes

PER SERVING
Calories 318
Total Fat 11.5 g
 Saturated Fat 3.0 g
 Trans Fat 0.0 g
 Polyunsaturated Fat 2.5 g
 Monounsaturated Fat 5.0 g
Cholesterol 10 mg
Sodium 386 mg
Carbohydrates 43 g
 Fiber 6 g
 Sugars 8 g
Protein 14 g
Dietary Exchanges
 2½ starch, 2 vegetable,
 1 lean meat, 1 fat

Layers of highly flavored ingredients ensure that every bite of this dish will explode with great taste.

- **6 ounces dried whole-grain penne (about 2¼ cups)**
- **1 teaspoon olive oil and 2 teaspoons olive oil, divided use**
- **1 cup finely chopped onion**
- **2 teaspoons bottled minced garlic or 4 medium garlic cloves, minced**
- **1 14.5-ounce can no-salt-added diced tomatoes, undrained**
- **¼ cup chopped fresh basil (about ⅔ ounce) or 1 tablespoon dried, crumbled**
- **1 tablespoon chopped fresh oregano or 1 teaspoon dried, crumbled**
- **1 teaspoon sugar**
- **¼ cup pine nuts, dry-roasted**
- **3 ounces crumbled low-fat feta cheese (about ¾ cup)**

Prepare the pasta using the package directions, omitting the salt. Drain well in a colander.

Meanwhile, in a medium saucepan, heat 1 teaspoon oil over medium-high heat, swirling to coat the bottom. Cook the onion for 3 minutes, or until soft, stirring frequently.

Stir in the garlic. Cook for 15 seconds, stirring constantly.

Stir in the tomatoes with liquid, basil and oregano if using dried, and sugar. Bring to a simmer. Reduce the heat and simmer for 15 minutes, or until the mixture is slightly thickened. Remove from the heat.

If using fresh basil and oregano, stir them into the tomato mixture. Stir in the pine nuts and remaining 2 teaspoons oil.

Pour the pasta onto a platter. Sprinkle with the feta. Mound the tomato mixture on top.

peanut pasta and vegetables

SERVES 4
1⅓ cups per serving

PREPARATION TIME
10 minutes

COOKING TIME
15 to 17 minutes

PER SERVING
Calories 352
Total Fat 11.5 g
  Saturated Fat 2.0 g
  Trans Fat 0.0 g
  Polyunsaturated Fat 3.5 g
  Monounsaturated Fat 5.5 g
Cholesterol 0 mg
Sodium 282 mg
Carbohydrates 52 g
  Fiber 9 g
  Sugars 8 g
Protein 14 g
Dietary Exchanges
  3½ starch, ½ lean meat,
  1½ fat

Kids will love this dish because of the creamy peanut sauce. Parents will love that the kids are eating whole-grain pasta.

8   ounces dried whole-grain spaghetti
6   ounces broccoli slaw mix (about 3 cups)
¼   cup creamy peanut butter
    (lowest sodium available)
3   tablespoons plain rice vinegar
2   tablespoons soy sauce (lowest sodium available)
1   tablespoon sugar
½   teaspoon bottled minced garlic or 1 medium garlic
    clove, minced
⅛   teaspoon cayenne
¼   cup chopped fresh basil (about ⅔ ounce) or
    snipped fresh cilantro
2   tablespoons chopped peanuts, dry-roasted

Prepare the pasta using the package directions, omitting the salt and adding the slaw mix during the last 1 minute of cooking time. Set aside ⅓ cup of the cooking liquid. Drain the pasta mixture well in a colander.

Meanwhile, in a large bowl, whisk together the peanut butter, vinegar, soy sauce, sugar, garlic, and cayenne.

Add the hot pasta mixture to the peanut butter mixture, stirring to coat. If the sauce is too thick, stir in the reserved cooking liquid 1 tablespoon at a time until creamy. Stir in the basil. Sprinkle with the peanuts.

COOK'S TIP
If you can't find broccoli slaw, you can use the same amount of any other type of refrigerated slaw mix that's available.

creamy green rice and black beans

SERVES 4
1¼ cups per serving

PREPARATION TIME
7 minutes

COOKING TIME
15 minutes

PER SERVING
Calories 218
Total Fat 1.0 g
 Saturated Fat 0.0 g
 Trans Fat 0.0 g
 Polyunsaturated Fat 0.5 g
 Monounsaturated Fat 0.5 g
Cholesterol 0 mg
Sodium 176 mg
Carbohydrates 40 g
 Fiber 7 g
 Sugars 5 g
Protein 12 g
Dietary Exchanges
 2½ starch, 1 vegetable,
 1 very lean meat

Combine a smooth spinach-based sauce, black beans, brown rice, and thick Greek yogurt for a hearty dinner. Serve it with sliced tomatoes.

1 poblano chile, quartered, seeds and ribs discarded if desired
½ cup coarsely chopped onion (yellow preferred)
1 medium garlic clove
3 to 4 ounces spinach (2 firmly packed cups)
¼ cup water (plus more as needed)
¼ teaspoon salt
1 15.5-ounce can no-salt-added black beans, rinsed and drained
10 ounces frozen cooked brown rice (about 2 cups)
½ cup fat-free plain Greek yogurt

In a large nonstick skillet, cook the poblano, onion, and garlic over medium-high heat for 8 to 10 minutes, or until the poblano is slightly blackened, stirring occasionally. Transfer to a food processor or blender.

Add the spinach, ¼ cup water, and salt. Process until smooth, adding more water 1 tablespoon at a time as needed, processing after each addition. Return the mixture to the skillet.

Stir in the beans. Cook over medium heat for 2 minutes, or until heated through.

Meanwhile, prepare the rice using the package directions.

Stir the yogurt into the poblano mixture. Stir in the rice.

COOK'S TIP ON POBLANO CHILES
Blackening poblanos in a skillet is an easy way to bring out the rich flavor of these long, triangular chiles.

bean-filled chiles rellenos

SERVES 4
1 stuffed pepper
per serving

PREPARATION TIME
10 minutes

COOKING TIME
13 to 15 minutes

MICROWAVE TIME
10 minutes

STANDING TIME
10 minutes

PER SERVING
Calories 276
Total Fat 3.0 g
  Saturated Fat 1.0 g
  Trans Fat 0.0 g
  Polyunsaturated Fat 0.5 g
  Monounsaturated Fat 1.0 g
Cholesterol 3 mg
Sodium 261 mg
Carbohydrates 47 g
  Fiber 13 g
  Sugars 14 g
Protein 18 g
Dietary Exchanges
  2 starch, 3 vegetable,
  1 very lean meat

Unlike many recipes for chiles rellenos, this one doesn't call for frying the stuffed chiles. Also, it uses canned beans without added salt to replace some of the usual cheese, providing protein and fiber while reducing the amount of saturated fat, cholesterol, and sodium.

4 **large poblano peppers**
   Cooking spray
1 **teaspoon olive oil**
1 **medium onion, chopped**
1 **tablespoon chili powder**
1 **teaspoon ground cumin**
1 **teaspoon bottled minced garlic or 2 medium garlic cloves, minced**
¼ **teaspoon salt**
2 **15.5-ounce cans no-salt-added pinto, small red, or black beans, rinsed and drained**
4 **medium Italian plum (Roma) tomatoes, chopped**
¼ **cup snipped fresh cilantro**
½ **cup shredded low-fat Cheddar cheese**
1 **medium lime, cut into 4 wedges**

In one side of each poblano pepper, cut a slit almost from end to end, being careful to keep the peppers intact. Transfer the peppers to a 9-inch square or round glass baking dish. Microwave, covered, on 100 percent power (high) for 10 minutes, or until tender. Remove from the microwave. Let stand, uncovered, for 10 minutes, or until cool enough to handle. Discard the ribs and seeds.

Meanwhile, preheat the broiler. Lightly spray a rimmed baking sheet with cooking spray. Set aside.

In a large nonstick skillet, heat the oil over medium-high heat, swirling to coat the bottom. Cook the onion for 3 minutes, or until soft, stirring frequently.

Stir in the chili powder, cumin, garlic, and salt. Cook for 1 minute, stirring frequently.

Stir in the beans and tomatoes. Cook for 4 to 5 minutes, or until the tomatoes are softened, stirring frequently. Stir in the cilantro.

Spoon 1 cup of the bean mixture into each pepper. Arrange the peppers in a single layer on the baking sheet. Sprinkle the peppers with the Cheddar.

Broil about 4 inches from the heat for 1 to 2 minutes, or until the Cheddar melts. Serve with the lime wedges to squeeze over the peppers.

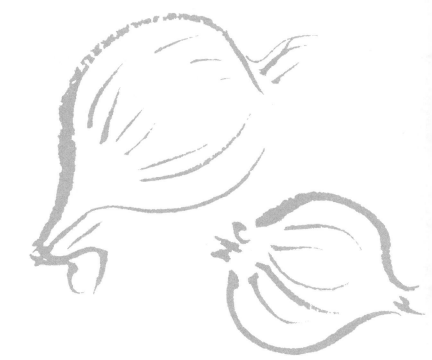

three-bean chili

SERVES 4
1¾ cups per serving

PREPARATION TIME
6 minutes

COOKING TIME
14 to 19 minutes

PER SERVING
Calories 411
Total Fat 2.0 g
  Saturated Fat 0.0 g
  Trans Fat 0.0 g
  Polyunsaturated Fat 0.5 g
  Monounsaturated Fat 0.0 g
Cholesterol 1 mg
Sodium 264 mg
Carbohydrates 71 g
  Fiber 16 g
  Sugars 15 g
Protein 23 g
Dietary Exchanges
  4 starch, 2 vegetable,
  1½ very lean meat

As more and more canned foods without added salt become available, such as the red kidney beans, pinto beans, and chickpeas (garbanzo beans) used here, it is getting easy to put healthy chili on the table in very little time, with very little effort, and with almost no cleanup involved.

1 **28-ounce can no-salt-added diced tomatoes, undrained**
1 **15.5-ounce can no-salt-added red kidney beans, rinsed and drained**
1 **15.5-ounce can no-salt-added pinto beans, rinsed and drained**
1 **15.5-ounce can no-salt-added chickpeas, rinsed and drained**
12 **ounces beer (light or nonalcoholic)**
2 **tablespoons chili powder**
2 **teaspoons ground cumin**
¼ **teaspoon salt**
½ **cup fat-free plain yogurt**
   Snipped fresh parsley or cilantro (optional)

In a large saucepan, stir together the tomatoes with liquid, beans, chickpeas, beer, chili powder, cumin, and salt. Bring to a boil over high heat. Reduce the heat and simmer for 10 to 15 minutes, or until the desired consistency. Ladle into bowls.

Top each serving with about 2 tablespoons yogurt. Sprinkle with the parsley.

white-bean veggie burgers

WITH AVOCADO TOPPING

Adding a topping of mashed avocado, sour cream, and fresh lime juice raises these bunless broiled burgers high above the norm.

SERVES 4
1 patty and
2 tablespoons topping
per serving

PREPARATION TIME
10 to 12 minutes

COOKING TIME
13 minutes

PER SERVING
Calories 359
Total Fat 12.5 g
  Saturated Fat 2.0 g
  Trans Fat 0.0 g
  Polyunsaturated Fat 1.5 g
  Monounsaturated Fat 8.5 g
Cholesterol 1 mg
Sodium 297 mg
Carbohydrates 46 g
  Fiber 13 g
  Sugars 8 g
Protein 17 g
Dietary Exchanges
  3 starch, 1 very lean meat,
  2 fat

Cooking spray
2 15.5-ounce cans no-salt-added navy beans, rinsed, drained, and coarsely mashed
1 4-ounce can chopped mild green chiles
⅓ cup uncooked quick-cooking oatmeal
2 large egg whites
1 tablespoon plus 1 teaspoon olive oil
2 teaspoons smoked paprika
1 teaspoon bottled minced garlic or 2 medium garlic cloves, minced
⅛ teaspoon salt and ⅛ teaspoon salt, divided use
1 medium avocado, mashed
2 tablespoons fat-free sour cream
1 tablespoon fresh lime juice

Preheat the broiler. Line a baking sheet with aluminum foil. Lightly spray the foil with cooking spray.

In a medium bowl, stir together the beans, chiles, oatmeal, egg whites, oil, paprika, garlic, and ⅛ teaspoon salt. Shape into 4 patties, each about 4 inches in diameter, or spoon 4 mounds of the mixture onto the baking sheet and flatten slightly to form patties. Lightly spray the tops with cooking spray.

Broil the patties about 4 inches from the heat for 8 minutes. Turn over. Lightly spray the tops with cooking spray. Broil for 5 minutes, or until lightly browned.

Meanwhile, in a small bowl, stir together the avocado, sour cream, lime juice, and remaining ⅛ teaspoon salt. Spoon the topping over the cooked patties.

COOK'S TIP
You can use a potato masher to coarsely mash the beans, or you might want to let the kids help you with the "squish" method. Pop the beans into an airtight plastic bag, squish them, squeeze them out, and then discard the bag—no potato masher, food processor, or blender required!

meatless tamale pie

SERVES 6
one 2 × 3-inch piece
per serving

PREPARATION TIME
8 minutes

COOKING TIME
32 minutes

PER SERVING
Calories 356
Total Fat 4.0 g
  Saturated Fat 0.5 g
  Trans Fat 0.0 g
  Polyunsaturated Fat 1.0 g
  Monounsaturated Fat 1.0 g
Cholesterol 0 mg
Sodium 421 mg
Carbohydrates 70 g
  Fiber 9 g
  Sugars 16 g
Protein 15 g
Dietary Exchanges
  4 starch, 2 vegetable,
  ½ very lean meat

Using packaged corn muffin mix for the casserole topping saves precious minutes in the kitchen.

Cooking spray
1 medium carrot, chopped
1 cup chopped onion
2 15.5-ounce cans no-salt-added kidney beans, rinsed and drained
1 12-ounce can no-salt-added whole-kernel corn, drained
1 8-ounce can no-salt-added tomato sauce
1 to 2 teaspoons chili powder
1 teaspoon ground cumin
1 8.5-ounce package corn muffin mix (lowest sodium available)
2 large egg whites
⅓ cup fat-free milk

Preheat the oven to 400°F. Lightly spray a 9-inch square glass baking dish and a large skillet with cooking spray. Set the dish aside.

In the skillet, cook the carrot and onion over medium-high heat for 5 minutes, or until the carrot is almost tender, stirring frequently.

Stir in the beans, corn, tomato sauce, chili powder, and cumin. Cook for 5 minutes, or until heated through, stirring occasionally.

Meanwhile, in a medium bowl, stir together the corn muffin mix, egg whites, and milk until smooth.

Spoon the carrot mixture into the baking dish. Spread the corn muffin batter over the mixture.

Bake for 20 minutes, or until the top is golden brown and a wooden toothpick inserted in the center comes out clean.

double-bean lettuce wraps

SERVES 4
2 wraps per serving

PREPARATION TIME
5 to 8 minutes

PER SERVING
Calories 120
Total Fat 0.0 g
  Saturated Fat 0.0 g
  Trans Fat 0.0 g
  Polyunsaturated Fat 0.0 g
  Monounsaturated Fat 0.0 g
Cholesterol 0 mg
Sodium 60 mg
Carbohydrates 22 g
  Fiber 6 g
  Sugars 4 g
Protein 8 g
Dietary Exchanges
  1½ starch, ½ very lean
  meat

Mild green chiles and cumin give these fiber-rich wraps a south-of-the-border flavor.

1	15.5-ounce can no-salt-added red kidney beans, rinsed, drained, and mashed
1	cup canned no-salt-added black beans, rinsed and drained
1	4-ounce can chopped green chiles, drained
1	teaspoon ground cumin
8	Bibb lettuce leaves
¼	cup Chunky Salsa (page 32) or commercial salsa (lowest sodium available)

In a medium bowl, stir together the beans, chiles, and cumin.

Spoon about ¼ cup bean mixture down the center of each lettuce leaf. Top with the salsa. Roll up jelly-roll style.

vegetarian couscous paella

SERVES 4
1¼ cups per serving

PREPARATION TIME
8 to 10 minutes

COOKING TIME
15 minutes

STANDING TIME
5 minutes

PER SERVING
Calories 315
Total Fat 1.0 g
 Saturated Fat 0.0 g
 Trans Fat 0.0 g
 Polyunsaturated Fat 0.5 g
 Monounsaturated Fat 0.0 g
Cholesterol 0 mg
Sodium 293 mg
Carbohydrates 65 g
 Fiber 12 g
 Sugars 4 g
Protein 14 g
Dietary Exchanges
 4 starch, 1 vegetable

Whole-wheat couscous replaces white rice in this meatless version of the traditional Spanish dish. Golden saffron gives it a special flavor as well as a lovely color, but if that spice isn't in your budget, you can substitute turmeric.

Cooking spray
1 small red onion, chopped
2 teaspoons bottled minced garlic or 4 medium garlic cloves, minced
1½ cups low-sodium vegetable broth
9 ounces frozen baby lima beans
3 to 4 ounces frozen green peas
¼ teaspoon salt
⅛ teaspoon powdered saffron or ½ teaspoon ground turmeric
⅛ teaspoon cayenne
1 cup uncooked whole-wheat couscous
1 medium tomato, chopped
¼ cup snipped fresh cilantro or parsley

Lightly spray a large saucepan with cooking spray. Cook the onion and garlic over medium-high heat for 3 minutes, or until the onion is soft, stirring frequently.

Stir in the broth, lima beans, peas, salt, saffron, and cayenne. Increase the heat to high and bring to a boil. Reduce the heat and simmer, covered, for 10 minutes, or until the lima beans are tender. Remove from the heat.

Stir in the couscous, tomato, and cilantro. Let stand, covered, for 5 minutes.

lentils

WITH GREEN BEANS, CARROTS, AND DRIED CURRANTS

SERVES 4
1¼ cups per serving

PREPARATION TIME
8 minutes

COOKING TIME
40 minutes

PER SERVING
Calories 246
Total Fat 1.0 g
  Saturated Fat 0.0 g
  Trans Fat 0.0 g
  Polyunsaturated Fat 0.5 g
  Monounsaturated Fat 0.0 g
Cholesterol 0 mg
Sodium 265 mg
Carbohydrates 48 g
  Fiber 16 g
  Sugars 16 g
Protein 15 g
Dietary Exchanges
  2 starch, ½ fruit,
  2 vegetable,
  1 very lean meat

Lentils are a powerhouse of fiber and other important nutrients. Unlike dried beans, they don't require soaking and long cooking times, making them great for busy cooks. Try them in this easy stovetop dish.

2 **cups water**
1 **cup dried green lentils, sorted for stones and shriveled lentils, rinsed, and drained**
1 **medium onion, chopped**
¼ **cup dried currants or raisins**
1 **teaspoon bottled minced garlic or 2 medium garlic cloves, minced**
½ **teaspoon curry powder**
¼ **teaspoon salt**
¼ **teaspoon pepper**
8 **ounces frozen cut green beans**
4 **medium carrots, cut crosswise into ½-inch slices**

In a large saucepan, bring the water, lentils, onion, currants, garlic, curry powder, salt, and pepper to a boil over high heat. Reduce the heat and simmer, covered, for 20 minutes.

Stir in the green beans and carrots. Return to a simmer and simmer, covered, for 15 to 20 minutes, or until the lentils and vegetables are tender, stirring occasionally.

barley and veggie stew
WITH MOZZARELLA AND PARMESAN

SERVES 4
1 cup per serving

PREPARATION TIME
15 minutes

COOKING TIME
16 minutes

PER SERVING
Calories 148
Total Fat 3.0 g
  Saturated Fat 1.0 g
  Trans Fat 0.0 g
  Polyunsaturated Fat 0.5 g
  Monounsaturated Fat 1.0 g
Cholesterol 9 mg
Sodium 400 mg
Carbohydrates 23 g
  Fiber 5 g
  Sugars 7 g
Protein 9 g
Dietary Exchanges
  1 starch, 2 vegetable,
  1 lean meat

Fresh tomatoes, green beans, and bell peppers give this stew great color, great texture, and—most important—great taste.

Cooking spray
2 medium red bell peppers, or 1 medium red bell pepper and 1 medium green bell pepper, cut into bite-size pieces
1 cup coarsely chopped onions (about 2 medium)
1 cup grape tomatoes, quartered
4 ounces green beans, trimmed and cut into 1-inch pieces
1½ cups water and ½ cup water, divided use
⅓ cup uncooked quick-cooking barley
1 teaspoon bottled minced garlic or 2 medium garlic cloves, minced
¼ cup chopped fresh basil (about ⅔ ounce)
1 teaspoon Louisiana hot sauce
¼ teaspoon salt
¾ cup shredded low-fat mozzarella cheese
1 tablespoon plus 1 teaspoon shredded or grated Parmesan cheese

Preheat the broiler. Line a rimmed baking sheet with aluminum foil. Lightly spray the foil with cooking spray.

Arrange the bell peppers, onions, tomatoes, and green beans in a single layer on the baking sheet. Lightly spray the vegetables with cooking spray.

Broil about 4 inches from the heat for 10 minutes, or until the edges are just beginning to lightly brown. Toss the vegetables, keeping them in a single layer. Broil for 5 minutes, or until richly browned on the edges.

Meanwhile, in a medium saucepan, bring 1½ cups water to a boil over high heat. Stir in the barley and garlic. Return to a boil. Reduce the heat and simmer, covered, for 10 to 12 minutes, or until the barley is tender. Don't drain.

Stir the broiled vegetables into the barley.

Pour the remaining ½ cup water onto the foil-lined baking sheet. Gently scrape the browned bits from the foil. Pour into the barley mixture.

Stir in the basil, hot sauce, and salt. Serve with the mozzarella and Parmesan sprinkled on top.

COOK'S TIP ON BARLEY
Substitute barley for pasta or rice to give dishes a new texture and "personality."

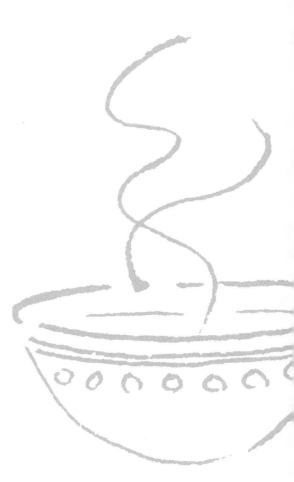

quinoa-vegetable patties

SERVES 4
1 patty, 1 tomato slice,
and 1 tablespoon yogurt
per serving

PREPARATION TIME
10 minutes

COOKING TIME
22 to 24 minutes

COOLING TIME
2 minutes

PER SERVING
Calories 183
Total Fat 5.5 g
 Saturated Fat 1.0 g
 Trans Fat 0.0 g
 Polyunsaturated Fat 1.0 g
 Monounsaturated Fat 2.5 g
Cholesterol 53 mg
Sodium 233 mg
Carbohydrates 27 g
 Fiber 5 g
 Sugars 4 g
Protein 9 g
Dietary Exchanges
 1½ starch, 1 vegetable,
 1 fat

Crisp on the outside but soft on the inside, the patties sit on sliced tomato and are topped with yogurt and dillweed.

½ **cup uncooked prerinsed quinoa**
8 **ounces frozen chopped broccoli (about 2½ cups)**
4 **ounces frozen cut green beans (about 1½ cups)**
½ **cup low-sodium vegetable broth**
¼ **cup finely chopped onion**
1 **teaspoon bottled minced garlic or 2 medium garlic cloves, minced**
⅓ **cup toasted wheat germ**
1 **large egg**
1 **teaspoon snipped fresh dillweed and 2 teaspoons snipped fresh dillweed, divided use**
½ **teaspoon red hot-pepper sauce**
¼ **teaspoon salt**
2 **teaspoons fresh lemon juice**
2 **teaspoons olive oil**
1 **medium tomato, cut into 4 slices**
¼ **cup fat-free plain yogurt**

Prepare the quinoa using the package directions, omitting the salt. Spread the quinoa on a large plate to cool for 2 minutes.

Meanwhile, in a large nonstick skillet, stir together the broccoli, green beans, broth, onion, and garlic. Cook over medium-high heat for 7 minutes, or until most of the broth has evaporated and the vegetables are tender.

While the broccoli mixture and quinoa cook, in a large bowl, whisk together the wheat germ, egg, 1 teaspoon dillweed, hot-pepper sauce, and salt. Set aside.

Transfer the cooked broccoli mixture to a food processor or blender. Add the lemon juice and process until smooth. Set aside. Stir the broccoli mixture and cooled quinoa into the wheat germ mixture.

Wipe the skillet with paper towels. Heat the oil over medium-high heat, swirling to coat the bottom. Form the vegetable mixture into four 4-inch patties. Cook for 4 minutes on each side, or until well browned. Serve each patty on a tomato slice. Top with the yogurt and remaining 2 teaspoons dillweed.

chickpeas and quinoa
WITH MANGO CHUTNEY

SERVES 4
1 cup quinoa and
¾ cup chickpea topping
per serving

PREPARATION TIME
11 minutes

COOKING TIME
16 to 17 minutes

STANDING TIME
5 minutes

PER SERVING
Calories 329
Total Fat 4.5 g
  Saturated Fat 0.5 g
  Trans Fat 0.0 g
  Polyunsaturated Fat 1.5 g
  Monounsaturated Fat 1.5 g
Cholesterol 0 mg
Sodium 357 mg
Carbohydrates 59 g
  Fiber 9 g
  Sugars 9 g
Protein 13 g
Dietary Exchanges
  3½ starch, 1 vegetable,
  1 very lean meat

Rather than being served as a condiment, tangy-sweet mango chutney is cooked along with the other distinctive ingredients in this Indian dish.

1 **cup uncooked prerinsed quinoa**
1 **teaspoon olive oil**
¾ **cup chopped onion**
1 **teaspoon grated peeled gingerroot**
1 **15.5-ounce can no-salt-added chickpeas, rinsed and drained**
1 **14.5-ounce can no-salt-added chopped tomatoes, undrained**
2 **tablespoons mango chutney (lowest sodium available)**
¾ **teaspoon curry powder**
½ **teaspoon ground cumin**
½ **teaspoon salt**
2 **medium green onions, chopped**
1 **medium lemon, cut into 4 wedges**

Prepare the quinoa using the package directions, omitting the salt. Remove from the heat. Fluff the quinoa with a fork. Let stand, covered, for 5 minutes.

Meanwhile, in a medium saucepan, heat the oil over medium-high heat, swirling to coat the bottom. Cook the onion and gingerroot for 3 minutes, or until the onion is soft, stirring frequently.

Stir in the chickpeas, tomatoes with liquid, chutney, curry powder, cumin, and salt. Cook for 5 minutes, or until heated through, stirring frequently.

Spoon the quinoa onto plates. Top with the chickpea mixture. Sprinkle with the green onions. Squeeze a lemon wedge over each serving.

COOK'S TIP ON QUINOA
Quinoa (KEEN-wah), a high-protein, calcium-rich grain from South America, has a wonderful crunchy texture and subtle nutty taste. The grains are covered with a bitter coating called saponin. If you didn't buy prerinsed quinoa, put it in a fine-mesh strainer and rinse it under cold running water for 1 to 2 minutes to remove all the bitterness.

no-yolk egg salad pita sandwiches

SERVES 4
1 sandwich per serving

PREPARATION TIME
10 minutes

COOKING TIME
17 minutes

STANDING TIME
3 minutes

PER SERVING
Calories 157
Total Fat 4.5 g
    Saturated Fat 0.5 g
    Trans Fat 0.0 g
    Polyunsaturated Fat 3.0 g
    Monounsaturated Fat 1.0 g
Cholesterol 5 mg
Sodium 447 mg
Carbohydrates 22 g
    Fiber 4 g
    Sugars 2 g
Protein 9 g
Dietary Exchanges
    1½ starch, 1 lean meat

This yolk-free pita sandwich filling gets its rich yellow color from mustard and turmeric instead of egg yolks, with celery and bell pepper providing crunch.

  6 **large eggs**
  ¼ **cup light mayonnaise**
  1 **medium green onion or ¼ medium shallot, finely chopped**
  1 **medium rib of celery, finely chopped**
  ½ **medium red bell pepper, finely chopped**
  1 **tablespoon yellow mustard (lowest sodium available)**
  ¼ **teaspoon ground turmeric**
  ¼ **to ½ teaspoon paprika**
  ¼ **teaspoon pepper**
  2 **6-inch whole-grain pita pockets, halved**
 24 **baby spinach leaves**

Put the eggs in a single layer in a large saucepan. Cover with cold water by 1 inch. Bring to a rolling boil, covered, over high heat. Remove from the heat. Let stand, covered, for 15 minutes. Drain. Immediately cover with cold water. Let stand for about 3 minutes, or until cool enough to handle. Peel the eggs. Cut each in half, discarding the yolks. Chop the egg whites.

Meanwhile, in a small bowl, stir together the mayonnaise, green onion, celery, bell pepper, mustard, turmeric, paprika, and pepper. Set aside.

Gently stir the egg whites into the mayonnaise mixture.

Line each pita half with 6 spinach leaves. Spoon the egg salad into the pita halves.

COOK'S TIP ON HARD-COOKED EGGS

You may know them as "hard-boiled" eggs, but "hard-cooked" actually is the accurate term. The cooking water does indeed need to come to a rolling boil, but as soon as that stage is reached, the pot of eggs is removed from the heat and the eggs sit in the hot water to cook. This method helps prevent rubbery eggs with green rings around the yolks.

To peel hard-cooked eggs, roll them on a flat surface, pressing gently until they have a fine network of lines all over the surface. Holding one egg at a time under cold running water (so the bits of shell will rinse off), peel from the larger end.

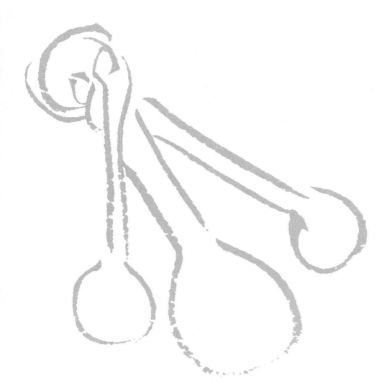

cheddar and vegetable crustless quiche

SERVES 6
1 wedge per serving

PREPARATION TIME
12 minutes

COOKING TIME
40 to 45 minutes

STANDING TIME
5 minutes

PER SERVING
Calories 119
Total Fat 4.0 g
  Saturated Fat 1.5 g
  Trans Fat 0.0 g
  Polyunsaturated Fat 0.5 g
  Monounsaturated Fat 1.5 g
Cholesterol 110 mg
Sodium 257 mg
Carbohydrates 10 g
  Fiber 1 g
  Sugars 3 g
Protein 11 g
Dietary Exchanges
  ½ starch, 1½ lean meat

Whether you serve this quiche for a weekend brunch or a weeknight dinner, you'll appreciate the simple preparation. Pair it with Double-Tomato Soup (page 45) for a lovely color contrast.

Cooking spray
3 large eggs
3 large egg whites
½ cup fat-free milk
2 tablespoons all-purpose flour
¼ teaspoon dried thyme, crumbled
⅛ teaspoon salt
⅛ teaspoon pepper
1 cup shredded low-fat sharp Cheddar cheese
1 cup bottled roasted red bell peppers, drained, patted dry, and chopped
¾ cup frozen whole-kernel corn, thawed
2 medium green onions, thinly sliced

Preheat the oven to 350°F. Lightly spray a 9-inch glass pie pan with cooking spray.

In a large bowl, whisk together the eggs, egg whites, milk, flour, thyme, salt, and pepper until smooth. Stir in the remaining ingredients. Pour into the pie pan.

Bake for 40 to 45 minutes, or until the top of the quiche is golden and the center is set (doesn't jiggle when the pan is lightly shaken). Let stand for 5 minutes before slicing.

greek omelet

SERVES 2
one-half omelet
per serving

PREPARATION TIME
10 minutes

COOKING TIME
5 minutes

PER SERVING
Calories 147
Total Fat 9.5 g
    Saturated Fat 2.5 g
    Trans Fat 0.0 g
    Polyunsaturated Fat 1.0 g
    Monounsaturated Fat 4.5 g
Cholesterol 213 mg
Sodium 278 mg
Carbohydrates 4 g
    Fiber 1 g
    Sugars 2 g
Protein 13 g
Dietary Exchanges
    2 lean meat, ½ fat

This savory omelet made with kalamata olives, feta cheese, and oregano combines classic flavors from Greece. Serve it with fresh fruit for breakfast or with Mediterranean Black Bean Salad (page 62) for dinner.

2 **large eggs**
2 **large egg whites**
1 **tablespoon finely chopped onion**
1 **tablespoon water**
¼ **teaspoon dried oregano, crumbled**
1 **teaspoon olive oil**
½ **cup shredded spinach**
¼ **cup chopped tomato**
1 **tablespoon finely chopped kalamata olives**
1 **tablespoon crumbled low-fat feta cheese**
2 **tablespoons fat-free plain Greek yogurt**
¼ **teaspoon pepper (coarsely ground preferred)**

In a medium bowl, whisk together the eggs, egg whites, onion, water, and oregano.

In a large nonstick skillet, heat the oil over medium heat, swirling to coat the bottom. Pour the egg mixture into the skillet, swirling to coat the bottom. Cook for 30 seconds. Using a spatula, carefully lift the cooked edge of the omelet and tilt the skillet so the uncooked portion flows under the edge. Cook until no runniness remains, repeating the lift-and-tilt procedure once or twice at other places along the edge if needed.

Sprinkle the spinach, tomato, olives, and feta over half of the omelet. Using a spatula, carefully fold the half with no filling over the other half.

Gently slide the omelet onto a dinner plate. Cut the omelet in half. Transfer one half to another plate. Top each serving with 1 tablespoon yogurt. Sprinkle with the pepper.

COOK'S TIP
Because the omelet cooks so fast, you'll want to have all your ingredients ready to go before you start.

green chile and tortilla casserole

SERVES 4
1 cup per serving

PREPARATION TIME
10 minutes

COOKING TIME
30 to 35 minutes

PER SERVING
Calories 170
Total Fat 4.5 g
  Saturated Fat 2.0 g
  Trans Fat 0.0 g
  Polyunsaturated Fat 0.5 g
  Monounsaturated Fat 1.5 g
Cholesterol 61 mg
Sodium 426 mg
Carbohydrates 18 g
  Fiber 3 g
  Sugars 6 g
Protein 14 g
Dietary Exchanges
  1 starch, 1 vegetable,
  1½ lean meat

This colorful layered casserole gets a slight tang from buttermilk.

    Cooking spray
6 6-inch corn tortillas, torn into bite-size pieces
1 4-ounce can chopped green chiles, drained
1 cup shredded low-fat Cheddar cheese
1 medium red bell pepper, chopped
4 medium green onions, thinly sliced
1 cup low-fat buttermilk
1 large whole egg
2 large egg whites

Preheat the oven to 325°F. Lightly spray a 9-inch square glass baking dish with cooking spray.

In the order listed, layer half of each of the following ingredients in the baking dish: tortillas, green chiles, Cheddar, bell pepper, and green onions. Repeat. Set aside.

In a small bowl, whisk together the buttermilk, egg, and egg whites. Gently pour over the casserole.

Bake for 30 to 35 minutes, or until a knife inserted near the center comes out clean.

lettuce bundles
WITH SWEET LIME SOY SAUCE

SERVES 4
3 lettuce bundles
per serving

PREPARATION TIME
15 minutes

COOKING TIME
5 minutes

PER SERVING
Calories 162
Total Fat 4.5 g
  Saturated Fat 0.5 g
  Trans Fat 0.0 g
  Polyunsaturated Fat 1.0 g
  Monounsaturated Fat 2.5 g
Cholesterol 0 mg
Sodium 279 mg
Carbohydrates 23 g
  Fiber 6 g
  Sugars 12 g
Protein 9 g
Dietary Exchanges
  2 vegetable, 1 other
  carbohydrate, 1 very lean
  meat, ½ fat

Different colors and textures are highlights of this easy entrée. Let the kids help with dinner by wrapping the lettuce leaves over the filling.

SAUCE
  3 **tablespoons sugar**
  3 **tablespoons fresh lime juice**
1½ **tablespoons soy sauce (lowest sodium available)**
  2 **teaspoons cider vinegar**
 ⅛ **teaspoon crushed red pepper flakes (optional)**

FILLING
  1 **teaspoon canola or corn oil**
  4 **ounces soy crumbles (ground meatless crumbles; about 1 cup), thawed if frozen**
1½ **cups finely shredded cabbage**
  1 **8-ounce can sliced water chestnuts, drained and finely chopped**
 ½ **cup finely chopped carrot**
 ⅓ **cup snipped fresh cilantro**
 ¼ **cup frozen green peas, thawed**
 ¼ **cup toasted sliced almonds**

12 **Boston or Bibb lettuce leaves**

In a small bowl, whisk together the sauce ingredients until the sugar is dissolved. Set aside.

In a large nonstick skillet, heat the oil over medium heat. Cook the crumbles for 4 minutes, or until heated through and beginning to brown, stirring occasionally. Remove from the heat.

Stir in the remaining filling ingredients. Don't reheat.

Put the lettuce leaves on a flat surface. Spoon about ⅓ cup filling into the center of each leaf. Top each with about 2 teaspoons sauce. Tightly roll up the leaves, jelly-roll style.

mushroom goulash

SERVES 6
1 heaping cup noodles
and ⅔ cup sauce
per serving

PREPARATION TIME
8 to 10 minutes

COOKING TIME
24 minutes

PER SERVING
Calories 302
Total Fat 2.5 g
  Saturated Fat 0.0 g
  Trans Fat 0.0 g
  Polyunsaturated Fat 0.5 g
  Monounsaturated Fat 1.0 g
Cholesterol 0 mg
Sodium 345 mg
Carbohydrates 53 g
  Fiber 10 g
  Sugars 6 g
Protein 19 g
Dietary Exchanges
  3 starch, 1 vegetable,
  1 very lean meat

This hearty goulash satisfies with robust flavors and a generous serving size. The yogurt makes a tangy alternative to sour cream in the sauce.

1 teaspoon olive oil
½ cup chopped onion
8 ounces presliced button mushrooms (about 2½ cups)
1 tablespoon sweet paprika
1 14.5-ounce can no-salt-added diced tomatoes, undrained
8 ounces soy crumbles (ground meatless crumbles; about 2 cups), thawed if frozen
½ teaspoon salt
½ teaspoon pepper
12 ounces dried whole-grain no-yolk noodles
½ cup fat-free plain yogurt
2 teaspoons all-purpose flour
2 tablespoons snipped fresh parsley

In a large nonstick skillet, heat the oil over medium-high heat, swirling to coat the bottom. Cook the onion for 3 minutes, or until soft, stirring frequently.

Stir in the mushrooms. Cook for 5 minutes, or until lightly browned, stirring occasionally.

Stir in the paprika. Cook for 1 minute, stirring constantly.

Stir in the tomatoes with liquid, soy crumbles, salt, and pepper. Bring to a boil, still over medium-high heat. Reduce the heat and simmer, covered, for 5 minutes. Increase the heat to medium high and bring to a gentle boil, uncovered. Gently boil for 5 minutes.

Meanwhile, prepare the noodles using the package directions, omitting the salt. Drain well in a colander.

In a small bowl, stir together the yogurt and flour. After the tomato mixture has gently boiled, stir in the yogurt mixture. Cook for 1 minute, still on medium high, stirring constantly. Serve the sauce over the noodles. Sprinkle with the parsley.

apricot-teriyaki tofu stir-fry

SERVES 4
1 cup tofu and vegetable
mixture and ½ cup rice
per serving

PREPARATION TIME
12 minutes

COOKING TIME
14 minutes

PER SERVING
Calories 263
Total Fat 10.0 g
  Saturated Fat 1.0 g
  Trans Fat 0.0 g
  Polyunsaturated Fat 3.0 g
  Monounsaturated Fat 5.0 g
Cholesterol 0 mg
Sodium 213 mg
Carbohydrates 36 g
  Fiber 5 g
  Sugars 13 g
Protein 8 g
Dietary Exchanges
  2 starch, 1 vegetable,
  1½ fat

A drizzle of sweet sauce with just a bit of fire tops cubes of tofu, brightly colored red bell pepper and asparagus, and crunchy almonds, all served over brown rice.

3 tablespoons all-fruit apricot spread
3 tablespoons teriyaki sauce
    (lowest sodium available)
2 tablespoons balsamic vinegar
⅛ teaspoon crushed red pepper flakes
10 ounces frozen cooked brown rice (about 2 cups)
1 tablespoon toasted sesame oil
1 medium red bell pepper, cut into thin strips
1 medium onion, cut into ½-inch wedges
6 ounces asparagus spears, trimmed and cut
    diagonally into 2-inch pieces
4 ounces light firm tofu, drained, patted dry, and cut
    into ½-inch cubes
½ cup sliced or slivered almonds (about 2 ounces),
    dry-roasted

In a small bowl, whisk together the apricot spread, teriyaki sauce, vinegar, and red pepper flakes. Set aside.

Prepare the rice using the package directions. Set aside.

Meanwhile, in a large nonstick skillet, heat the oil over medium-high heat, swirling to coat the bottom. Cook the bell pepper and onion for 2 minutes, stirring frequently.

Stir in the asparagus and tofu. Cook for 2 minutes, or until the asparagus is tender-crisp. Stir in the almonds.

Spoon the brown rice onto a platter. Top with the tofu mixture. Set aside.

In the same skillet, bring the apricot spread mixture to a boil over medium-high heat, scraping the bottom and side of the skillet to dislodge any browned bits and stirring constantly. Drizzle over the tofu mixture.

tofu parmesan

SERVES 4
2 tofu slices and
⅓ cup sauce
per serving

PREPARATION TIME
10 to 12 minutes

COOKING TIME
16 to 18 minutes

PER SERVING
Calories 169
Total Fat 7.0 g
  Saturated Fat 2.0 g
  Trans Fat 0.0 g
  Polyunsaturated Fat 0.5 g
  Monounsaturated Fat 3.5 g
Cholesterol 6 mg
Sodium 274 mg
Carbohydrates 13 g
  Fiber 2 g
  Sugars 4 g
Protein 13 g
Dietary Exchanges
  ½ starch, 1 vegetable,
  1½ lean meat, ½ fat

Parmesan cheese and panko crumbs make an irresistibly crisp crust for slices of tofu.

SAUCE

- 1 teaspoon olive oil
- ¼ cup diced onion
- ½ teaspoon bottled minced garlic or 1 medium garlic clove, minced
- 1 14.5-ounce can no-salt-added diced tomatoes, undrained
- ¼ teaspoon dried basil, crumbled
- ⅛ teaspoon salt

- 1 large egg white
- 2 tablespoons water
- ½ cup plain panko (Japanese bread crumbs)
- ¼ cup shredded or grated Parmesan cheese
- ½ teaspoon dried oregano, crumbled
- ⅛ teaspoon pepper
- 12 ounces light firm tofu, well drained, cut into 8 slices
- 1 teaspoon olive oil and 1 teaspoon olive oil, divided use
- ¼ cup grated low-fat mozzarella cheese

In a medium skillet, heat 1 teaspoon oil over medium-high heat, swirling to coat the bottom. Cook the onion for 2 minutes, or until almost soft, stirring frequently.

Stir in the garlic. Cook for 1 minute, stirring constantly.

Stir in the tomatoes with liquid, basil, and salt. Using a potato masher, mash the tomatoes to make the sauce almost smooth. Bring to a boil, still over medium-high heat. Reduce the heat and simmer for 10 minutes, or until the sauce is thickened. Cover to keep warm. Set aside.

Meanwhile, in a small shallow dish, whisk together the egg white and water.

In a medium shallow dish, stir together the panko, Parmesan, oregano, and pepper.

Put the dishes and a large plate in a row, assembly-line fashion. Dip 1 slice of tofu in the egg white mixture, turning to coat and letting any excess drip off. Dip in the panko mixture, turning to coat. Using your fingertips, gently press the panko mixture so it adheres to the tofu. Transfer to the plate. Repeat with the remaining tofu.

In a large nonstick skillet, heat 1 teaspoon oil over medium heat, swirling to coat the bottom. Cook half the tofu for 2 to 3 minutes on each side, or until the coating is well browned. Transfer to a separate large plate. Cover to keep warm. Repeat with the final 1 teaspoon oil and remaining tofu.

Arrange the tofu on plates. Top with the sauce. Sprinkle with the mozzarella.

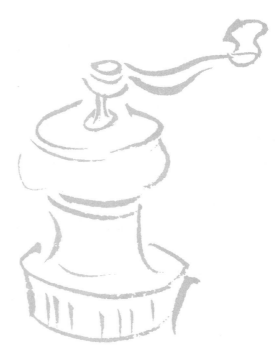

sesame tofu and vegetable stir-fry

SERVES 4
1 cup tofu and vegetable mixture and scant ½ cup rice per serving

PREPARATION TIME
15 minutes

COOKING TIME
8 to 10 minutes

PER SERVING
Calories 183
Total Fat 5.0 g
    Saturated Fat 0.5 g
    Trans Fat 0.0 g
    Polyunsaturated Fat 1.5 g
    Monounsaturated Fat 1.5 g
Cholesterol 0 mg
Sodium 264 mg
Carbohydrates 24 g
    Fiber 3 g
    Sugars 2 g
Protein 11 g
Dietary Exchanges
    1½ starch, 1 vegetable,
    1 lean meat

Lime juice adds such an enjoyable tart, fresh flavor that even people who shy away from tofu will love this all-in-one meal. Try Sherbet Parfaits (page 253) as a sweet finish to dinner.

2 tablespoons fresh lime juice
2 tablespoons soy sauce (lowest sodium available)
1 teaspoon cornstarch
⅛ teaspoon crushed red pepper flakes
10 ounces frozen cooked brown rice (about 2 cups)
2 teaspoons toasted sesame oil
2 teaspoons minced peeled gingerroot
1 teaspoon bottled minced garlic or 2 medium garlic cloves, minced
1 medium yellow bell pepper, cut into ¼-inch strips
2 medium green onions, cut into 1-inch pieces
12 ounces light firm tofu, well drained, patted dry, and cut into ½-inch cubes
6 ounces baby spinach (about 6 cups)
1 teaspoon sesame seeds

In a small bowl, whisk together the lime juice, soy sauce, cornstarch, and red pepper flakes until the cornstarch is dissolved. Set aside.

Prepare the rice using the package directions. Set aside.

Meanwhile, in a large nonstick skillet, heat the oil over medium-high heat, swirling to coat the bottom. Cook the gingerroot and garlic for 30 seconds, or until fragrant, stirring constantly.

Stir in the bell pepper and green onions. Cook for 2 to 3 minutes, or until tender-crisp, stirring constantly.

Stir in the tofu. Cook for 2 minutes, or until heated through, stirring frequently.

Stir in the lime juice mixture. Add half the spinach. Cook for 2 to 3 minutes, or until just wilted, stirring constantly. Repeat with the remaining spinach.

Spoon the rice onto a platter. Top with the tofu mixture. Sprinkle with the sesame seeds just before serving.

tempeh
WITH ASIAN SLAW

SERVES 4
3 ounces tempeh and
1 cup slaw
per serving

PREPARATION TIME
8 to 10 minutes

COOKING TIME
18 minutes

PER SERVING
Calories 214
Total Fat 8.0 g
  Saturated Fat 1.5 g
  Trans Fat 0.0 g
  Polyunsaturated Fat 3.0 g
  Monounsaturated Fat 3.0 g
Cholesterol 0 mg
Sodium 89 mg
Carbohydrates 19 g
  Fiber 10 g
  Sugars 4 g
Protein 20 g
Dietary Exchanges
  1 starch, 1 vegetable,
  2 lean meat

Orange juice spiked with Asian seasonings flavors both the protein-rich tempeh and the quickly warmed premade broccoli slaw mix in this dish. Serve it with fresh fruit on the side.

1   teaspoon toasted sesame oil
½   teaspoon bottled minced garlic or 1 medium garlic clove, minced
⅓   cup fresh orange juice (plus 1 to 2 tablespoons fresh orange juice or water as needed)
¼   cup plain rice vinegar
2   teaspoons soy sauce (lowest sodium available)
½   teaspoon ground ginger
12 ounces tempeh
10 ounces broccoli slaw mix (about 4 cups)
¼   cup sliced green onions

In a large nonstick skillet, heat the oil over medium heat, swirling to coat the bottom. Cook the garlic for 2 minutes, stirring frequently.

Stir in ⅓ cup orange juice, the vinegar, soy sauce, and ginger. Bring to a simmer, still over medium heat. Add the tempeh. Simmer, covered, for 10 minutes, turning once halfway through. Transfer the tempeh to a medium plate. Set aside.

If the tempeh absorbed most of the liquid, add the extra 1 to 2 tablespoons orange juice to the skillet. Add the broccoli slaw, stirring to coat. Cook for 4 minutes, or until the slaw is slightly wilted, stirring occasionally.

Meanwhile, cut the tempeh into thin strips.

Spoon the slaw onto plates. Top with the tempeh. Sprinkle with the green onions.

COOK'S TIP ON TEMPEH
Tempeh (TEHM-pay) is a firm piece of fermented soybeans with a nutty flavor and chewy texture. Sometimes grains, seeds, and nuts are added to vary the flavor. Tempeh contains as much protein as beef or chicken and more than tofu. You can slice tempeh, form it into patties, or crumble it, then bake, broil, grill, or stir-fry the pieces.

summer succotash

WITH CREAMY POLENTA

SERVES 4
1 cup vegetable mixture and scant ½ cup polenta per serving

PREPARATION TIME
12 to 15 minutes

COOKING TIME
13 to 15 minutes

PER SERVING
Calories 242
Total Fat 4.5 g
  Saturated Fat 1.5 g
  Trans Fat 0.0 g
  Polyunsaturated Fat 0.5 g
  Monounsaturated Fat 2.5 g
Cholesterol 4 mg
Sodium 372 mg
Carbohydrates 43 g
  Fiber 7 g
  Sugars 5 g
Protein 10 g
Dietary Exchanges
  3 starch, ½ fat

Fresh basil adds flavor and an enticing aroma to this fusion dish. While the succotash simmers, make the polenta, which adds a touch of Italy to a southern dish.

SUCCOTASH

- **2 teaspoons olive oil**
- **½ cup chopped onion**
- **½ cup chopped red bell pepper**
- **½ teaspoon bottled minced garlic or 1 medium garlic clove, minced**
- **10 ounces frozen baby lima beans, thawed**
- **1 cup frozen whole-kernel corn, thawed**
- **½ cup low-sodium vegetable broth**
- **¼ teaspoon salt**
- **⅛ teaspoon pepper**
- **2 medium Italian plum (Roma) tomatoes, chopped**
- **3 tablespoons snipped fresh basil**

POLENTA

- **2 cups low-sodium vegetable broth**
- **½ cup yellow cornmeal**
- **¼ cup shredded or grated Parmesan cheese**
- **⅛ teaspoon pepper**

In a large nonstick skillet, heat the oil over medium-high heat, swirling to coat the bottom. Cook the onion and bell pepper for 3 minutes, or until soft, stirring frequently.

Stir in the garlic. Cook for 1 minute, stirring frequently.

Stir in the beans, corn, ½ cup broth, salt, and pepper. Bring to a boil, still over medium-high heat. Reduce the heat and simmer, covered, for 4 to 5 minutes, or until the beans and corn are tender-crisp, stirring occasionally.

Stir in the tomatoes. Cook for 1 to 2 minutes, or until heated through. Remove from the heat. Stir in the basil.

Meanwhile, for the polenta, bring 2 cups broth to a boil over medium-high heat. Slowly whisk the cornmeal into the broth, whisking constantly. Cook for 1 to 2 minutes, or until the polenta is very thick, stirring (not whisking) constantly. Remove from the heat.

Stir in the Parmesan and pepper. Spoon into shallow bowls. Spoon the succotash over the polenta.

COOK'S TIP
Use the polenta part of this recipe to serve with entrées ranging from roasted chicken to beef stew.

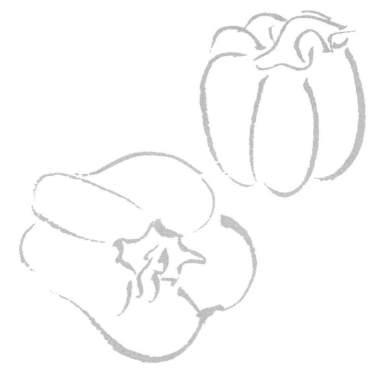

vegetables and side dishes

roasted asparagus and mushrooms

WITH ROSEMARY

SERVES 4
¾ cup per serving

PREPARATION TIME
10 minutes

COOKING TIME
10 minutes

PER SERVING
Calories 58
Total Fat 2.5 g
  Saturated Fat 0.5 g
  Trans Fat 0.0 g
  Polyunsaturated Fat 0.5 g
  Monounsaturated Fat 1.5 g
Cholesterol 0 mg
Sodium 77 mg
Carbohydrates 7 g
  Fiber 3 g
  Sugars 3 g
Protein 4 g
Dietary Exchanges
  1 vegetable, ½ fat

Roasting vegetables brings out their natural sugars and gives them a lightly sweet flavor, well complemented by fresh rosemary.

1   **pound fresh asparagus, trimmed**
8   **ounces shiitake or button mushrooms, stems discarded if shiitake**
2   **teaspoons olive oil**
½   **teaspoon finely snipped fresh rosemary or ¼ teaspoon dried, crushed**
½   **teaspoon garlic powder**
⅛   **teaspoon salt**
    Pepper to taste

Preheat the oven to 500°F.

Place the asparagus and mushrooms in a large shallow dish. Drizzle with the oil. Sprinkle with the rosemary, garlic powder, salt, and pepper. Turn the asparagus and mushrooms gently to coat. Arrange them in a single layer on a baking sheet.

Roast for 10 minutes, or until the asparagus is tender-crisp.

toasted barley pilaf

SERVES 4
½ cup per serving

PREPARATION TIME
6 minutes

COOKING TIME
32 minutes

PER SERVING

Calories 183
Total Fat 0.5 g
  Saturated Fat 0.0 g
  Trans Fat 0.0 g
  Polyunsaturated Fat 0.5 g
  Monounsaturated Fat 0.0 g
Cholesterol 0 mg
Sodium 117 mg
Carbohydrates 39 g
  Fiber 8 g
  Sugars 1 g
Protein 6 g
Dietary Exchanges
  2½ starch

Browning barley before cooking it provides a nutty flavor, making this dish taste similar to brown rice pilaf. Try this delightfully chewy side with Skillet Chicken with Dried Berries (page 107) or Pepper-Rubbed Beef with Mushroom Sauce (page 142) tonight.

1 cup uncooked pearl barley
2 cups fat-free, low-sodium chicken broth
½ cup sliced celery
¼ teaspoon finely snipped fresh rosemary or ⅛ teaspoon dried, crushed
⅛ teaspoon salt
⅛ teaspoon pepper

In a large heavy skillet, cook the barley over medium heat for 10 minutes, or until lightly toasted, stirring occasionally.

Slowly stir in the broth. Stir in the remaining ingredients. Increase the heat to high and bring to a boil. Reduce the heat and simmer, covered, for 20 minutes, or until the liquid is absorbed.

broccoli
WITH CREAMY DIJON SAUCE

SERVES 4
2/3 cup per serving

PREPARATION TIME
3 minutes

COOKING TIME
10 minutes

PER SERVING
Calories 40
Total Fat 0.5 g
  Saturated Fat 0.0 g
  Trans Fat 0.0 g
  Polyunsaturated Fat 0.0 g
  Monounsaturated Fat 0.0 g
Cholesterol 1 mg
Sodium 88 mg
Carbohydrates 7 g
  Fiber 2 g
  Sugars 2 g
Protein 3 g
Dietary Exchanges
  1 vegetable

RED POTATOES WITH
CREAMY DIJON SAUCE

Calories 96
Total Fat 0.5 g
  Saturated Fat 0.0 g
  Trans Fat 0.0 g
  Polyunsaturated Fat 0.0 g
  Monounsaturated Fat 0.0 g
Cholesterol 1 mg
Sodium 72 mg
Carbohydrates 21 g
  Fiber 2 g
  Sugars 2 g
Protein 3 g
Dietary Exchanges
  1½ starch

Chicken broth replaces water for boiling the broccoli and then becomes the base for a creamy mustard sauce. Both the broccoli and the sauce are cooked in the same saucepan, making cleanup a snap.

½ **cup fat-free, low-sodium chicken broth (plus more as needed)**
½ **teaspoon dried thyme, crumbled**
8 **ounces broccoli florets (about 3 cups)**
2 **tablespoons fat-free sour cream**
2 **teaspoons all-purpose flour**
2 **teaspoons Dijon mustard (lowest sodium available)**

In a medium saucepan, bring ½ cup broth and the thyme to a boil over high heat. Stir in the broccoli. Return to a boil. Reduce the heat and simmer, covered, for 5 minutes, or until the broccoli is tender-crisp. Using a slotted spoon, transfer the broccoli to a large plate, leaving the cooking liquid in the pan. Cover the broccoli to keep warm. Set aside.

Meanwhile, in a small bowl, whisk together the sour cream, flour, and mustard. Whisk the mixture into the broth. Cook over medium heat for 3 minutes, whisking constantly. Don't let the sauce boil. If the sauce is too thick, whisk in more broth, 1 tablespoon at a time, until the desired consistency. Remove the pan from the heat.

Add the broccoli to the sauce, stirring gently to coat.

red potatoes with creamy dijon sauce

Prepare the recipe as directed above, but substitute 1 pound small red potatoes, cut into bite-size pieces, for the broccoli and ¼ teaspoon dried dillweed, crumbled, for the thyme. Cook the potatoes for 10 to 15 minutes, or until tender.

brussels sprouts
WITH ORANGE-SESAME SAUCE

SERVES 4
⅔ cup per serving

PREPARATION TIME
5 minutes

COOKING TIME
11 to 13 minutes

MICROWAVE TIME
30 seconds

PER SERVING
Calories 38
Total Fat 1.0 g
  Saturated Fat 0.0 g
  Trans Fat 0.0 g
  Polyunsaturated Fat 0.5 g
  Monounsaturated Fat 0.5 g
Cholesterol 0 mg
Sodium 87 mg
Carbohydrates 7 g
  Fiber 3 g
  Sugars 2 g
Protein 3 g
Dietary Exchanges
  1 vegetable

The orange sauce in this recipe is super quick to make and tastes super delicious as well. Once you taste how good it is, you'll also want to serve it over other vegetables, such as broccoli, carrots, or snow peas.

10 **ounces frozen brussels sprouts**
SAUCE
 2 **teaspoons water**
 2 **teaspoons frozen orange juice concentrate**
 1 **teaspoon light tub margarine**
 ¼ **teaspoon sesame seeds, dry-roasted if desired**
 ⅛ **teaspoon salt**

Prepare the brussels sprouts using the package directions. Drain well in a colander. Transfer to a serving bowl.

Meanwhile, in a 1-cup glass measuring cup, micro-wave the water, orange juice concentrate, margarine, sesame seeds, and salt on 100 percent power (high) for 30 seconds, or until the orange juice thaws and the margarine is melted. Stir. Set aside.

When the brussels sprouts are done, pour the sauce over them, tossing to coat.

gingered bulgur and dried apricots

Fresh gingerroot, dried apricots, and ground cinnamon provide a flavor boost for fiber-rich bulgur.

2 **cups water**
1 **cup instant, or fine-grain, bulgur**
¼ **cup chopped dried apricots or mixed dried fruit bits**
1 **tablespoon grated peeled gingerroot**
⅛ **teaspoon salt**
¼ **teaspoon ground cinnamon**

In a medium saucepan, stir together all the ingredients. Bring to a boil over high heat. Reduce the heat and simmer, covered, for 5 minutes, or until the liquid is absorbed.

cauliflower
WITH PEANUT DIPPING SAUCE

SERVES 4
2/3 cup cauliflower and
1 tablespoon sauce
per serving

PREPARATION TIME
10 minutes

COOKING TIME
9 minutes

PER SERVING
Calories 55
Total Fat 2.5 g
  Saturated Fat 0.5 g
  Trans Fat 0.0 g
  Polyunsaturated Fat 0.5 g
  Monounsaturated Fat 1.0 g
Cholesterol 0 mg
Sodium 44 mg
Carbohydrates 8 g
  Fiber 2 g
  Sugars 4 g
Protein 3 g
Dietary Exchanges
  1 vegetable, ½ fat

Enjoy a quick trip to Indonesia, courtesy of the exciting flavor combination of peanut butter, apple juice, lime, and curry powder in this dipping sauce.

½ **cup water**
3 **cups cauliflower florets**
4½ **tablespoons unsweetened apple juice**
1 **tablespoon creamy peanut butter (lowest sodium available)**
½ **teaspoon grated lime zest**
1 **teaspoon fresh lime juice**
½ **teaspoon bottled minced garlic or 1 medium garlic clove, minced**
¼ **teaspoon curry powder**
⅛ **teaspoon cornstarch**
Dash of cayenne

In a medium saucepan, bring the water to a boil over medium-high heat. Boil the cauliflower, covered, for 8 minutes, or until tender-crisp. Drain well in a colander.

Meanwhile, in a small saucepan, stir together the remaining ingredients. Cook over medium-high heat for 5 to 7 minutes, or until the desired consistency, stirring occasionally. Serve the cauliflower with the dipping sauce.

colorful lemon couscous

SERVES 6
½ cup per serving

PREPARATION TIME
8 minutes

COOKING TIME
8 minutes

STANDING TIME
5 minutes

PER SERVING
Calories 150
Total Fat 0.5 g
  Saturated Fat 0.0 g
  Trans Fat 0.0 g
  Polyunsaturated Fat 0.5 g
  Monounsaturated Fat 0.0 g
Cholesterol 0 mg
Sodium 59 mg
Carbohydrates 32 g
  Fiber 5 g
  Sugars 1 g
Protein 6 g
Dietary Exchanges
  2 starch

Serve this grain-based dish along with steamed spinach and Dilled Albacore Cakes (page 94) or Coriander-Coated Chicken (page 113) for a nutritious meal.

Cooking spray
1 small green bell pepper, chopped
1 small red or yellow bell pepper, chopped
1 teaspoon bottled minced garlic or 2 medium garlic cloves, minced
1 cup fat-free, low-sodium chicken broth
⅛ teaspoon salt
1 cup uncooked whole-wheat couscous
1 teaspoon finely grated lemon zest
1 tablespoon fresh lemon juice

Lightly spray a medium saucepan with cooking spray. Cook the bell peppers and garlic over medium-high heat for 5 minutes, or until tender, stirring frequently.

Stir in the broth and salt. Increase the heat to high and bring to a boil. Stir in the couscous, lemon zest, and lemon juice. Remove from the heat.

Let stand, covered, for 5 minutes, or until the liquid is absorbed. Just before serving, fluff with a fork.

green bean toss-up

SERVES 4
¾ cup per serving

PREPARATION TIME
5 minutes

COOKING TIME
5 to 8 minutes

PER SERVING

Calories 62
Total Fat 4.0 g
  Saturated Fat 0.5 g
  Trans Fat 0.0 g
  Polyunsaturated Fat 0.5 g
  Monounsaturated Fat 2.5 g
Cholesterol 0 mg
Sodium 133 mg
Carbohydrates 7 g
  Fiber 3 g
  Sugars 3 g
Protein 2 g
Dietary Exchanges
  1 vegetable, 1 fat

Kick up the flavor of the green beans in this veggie toss-up by seasoning them with a few high-intensity ingredients. Serve the beans as a side with Crunchy Fish Nuggets with Lemon Tartar Sauce (page 76).

12 **ounces green beans, trimmed**
1 **tablespoon Dijon mustard (lowest sodium available)**
1 **tablespoon olive oil (extra-virgin preferred)**
2 **teaspoons Louisiana hot sauce (lowest sodium available)**
1 **tablespoon snipped fresh parsley**

In a medium saucepan, steam the beans for 4 to 7 minutes, or until tender-crisp. Drain well.

Meanwhile, in a medium bowl, stir together the mustard, oil, and hot sauce. Add the beans, stirring to coat. Stir in the parsley.

citrus kale

WITH DRIED CRANBERRIES

SERVES 4
½ cup per serving

PREPARATION TIME
7 minutes

COOKING TIME
23 to 25 minutes

PER SERVING

Calories 75
Total Fat 1.5 g
  Saturated Fat 0.0 g
  Trans Fat 0.0 g
  Polyunsaturated Fat 0.5 g
  Monounsaturated Fat 1.0 g
Cholesterol 0 mg
Sodium 99 mg
Carbohydrates 15 g
  Fiber 2 g
  Sugars 8 g
Protein 2 g
Dietary Exchanges
  ½ fruit, 1 vegetable, ½ fat

Balsamic vinegar and a splash of orange juice really jazz up the mild flavor of kale. So easy and so good!

3 **quarts water**
8 **ounces chopped kale, any large stems discarded (about 5 cups)**
1 **teaspoon olive oil**
¼ **cup sweetened dried cranberries**
2 **tablespoons balsamic vinegar**
1 **teaspoon bottled minced garlic or 2 medium garlic cloves, minced**
⅛ **teaspoon salt**
2 **tablespoons fresh orange juice**
1 **teaspoon grated orange zest**

In a stockpot, bring the water to a boil, covered, over high heat. Cook the kale, uncovered, for 8 minutes, or until softened, stirring occasionally. Transfer to a colander. Immediately run under cold water for 1 to 2 minutes, or until cool. Using the back of a large spoon, gently press on the kale to remove the moisture.

In a large skillet, heat the oil over medium-high heat, swirling to coat the bottom. Cook the kale, cranberries, vinegar, garlic, and salt for 2 to 3 minutes, or until heated through, stirring frequently. Remove from the heat.

Stir in the orange juice and zest.

COOK'S TIP
Look for packages of prewashed and prechopped kale (and other types of greens, such as the collard greens for Spicy Penne with Greens and Beans, page 174) in the produce section of your supermarket. If bought loose, the greens need to be stemmed, then rinsed several times before they're clean and ready to use, so buying packaged greens saves lots of time.

COOK'S TIP ON BOILING WATER
Liquid will come to a boil faster if you cover the pot.

german-style noodles

PREPARATION TIME
10 to 12 minutes

COOKING TIME
15 to 18 minutes

PER SERVING

Calories 115
Total Fat 0.5 g
  Saturated Fat 0.0 g
  Trans Fat 0.0 g
  Polyunsaturated Fat 0.0 g
  Monounsaturated Fat 0.0 g
Cholesterol 3 mg
Sodium 136 mg
Carbohydrates 23 g
  Fiber 2 g
  Sugars 3 g
Protein 4 g
Dietary Exchanges
  1½ starch

Cabbage, carrots, and caraway seeds enhance the noodles in this one-pan stovetop dish. Try it with Sliced Sirloin with Leek Sauce (page 146) or broiled lean pork chops.

  6 **cups water**
  4 **ounces dried medium no-yolk noodles (3 heaping cups)**
  ½ **cup sliced carrots**
  1 **cup chopped cabbage**
  ½ **cup fat-free sour cream**
  2 **medium green onions, sliced**
  ½ **teaspoon caraway seeds**
  ¼ **teaspoon salt**
  ⅛ **teaspoon pepper**

In a large saucepan, bring the water to a boil, covered, over high heat. Stir in the noodles and carrots. Reduce the heat and boil gently, uncovered, for 5 minutes.

Stir in the cabbage. Cook for 3 to 5 minutes, or until the noodles are tender. Drain the mixture well in a colander. Return to the pan.

Stir in the remaining ingredients. Reduce the heat to low and cook for 1 to 2 minutes, or until heated through (don't let the mixture come to a boil).

bow tie pasta

WITH SPINACH AND RADICCHIO

SERVES 6
heaping 2/3 cup
per serving

PREPARATION TIME
10 minutes

COOKING TIME
10 to 12 minutes

PER SERVING
Calories 73
Total Fat 2.0 g
    Saturated Fat 0.5 g
    Trans Fat 0.0 g
    Polyunsaturated Fat 0.0 g
    Monounsaturated Fat 1.0 g
Cholesterol 2 mg
Sodium 67 mg
Carbohydrates 11 g
    Fiber 2 g
    Sugars 1 g
Protein 3 g
Dietary Exchanges
    ½ starch, ½ fat

Keep this colorful recipe in mind for a celebratory dinner side dish or pair it with a cup of soup for a satisfying lunch.

2   **cups dried whole-grain bow-tie pasta or medium shell pasta**
1   **teaspoon olive oil**
½   **teaspoon bottled minced garlic or 1 medium garlic clove, minced**
1   **to 2 tablespoons balsamic vinegar**
2   **ounces spinach, torn into bite-size pieces (about 2 cups)**
1   **cup torn radicchio**
¼   **cup shredded or grated Parmesan cheese**

Prepare the pasta using the package directions, omitting the salt. Drain well in a colander.

Meanwhile, in a small skillet, heat the oil over medium heat, swirling to coat the bottom. Cook the garlic for 1 minute, or until tender, stirring occasionally.

Stir in the vinegar. Remove from the heat.

Put the spinach and radicchio in a large bowl. Add the pasta. Pour the garlic mixture over all, stirring to coat. Sprinkle with the Parmesan.

angel hair pasta
WITH RED PEPPER AND TOMATO SAUCE

SERVES 4
½ cup pasta and
¼ cup sauce
per serving

PREPARATION TIME
5 minutes

COOKING TIME
10 to 12 minutes

PER SERVING
Calories 120
Total Fat 1.0 g
    Saturated Fat 0.0 g
    Trans Fat 0.0 g
    Polyunsaturated Fat 0.5 g
    Monounsaturated Fat 0.5 g
Cholesterol 0 mg
Sodium 162 mg
Carbohydrates 24 g
    Fiber 4 g
    Sugars 3 g
Protein 5 g
Dietary Exchanges
    1½ starch, 1 vegetable

Pair this pasta with Baked Chicken with Crunchy Basil-Parmesan Pesto (page 103) for an Italian feast tonight!

  4 **ounces uncooked whole-grain angel hair pasta**
SAUCE
  1 **large red bell pepper, chopped**
  ⅔ **cup fat-free, low-sodium chicken broth**
  ¼ **teaspoon salt**
  ⅛ **to ¼ teaspoon pepper**
     Dash of cayenne
  1 **tablespoon plus 1 teaspoon no-salt-added tomato paste**

Prepare the pasta using the package directions, omitting the salt. Drain well in a colander. Transfer to a large bowl.

Meanwhile, in a small saucepan, stir together the sauce ingredients except the tomato paste. Bring to a boil over high heat. Reduce the heat and simmer, covered, for 5 minutes, or until the bell pepper is tender.

Transfer the sauce to a food processor or blender. Add the tomato paste. Process until smooth. Pour over the pasta, stirring to coat.

sesame pasta and vegetables

SERVES 4
1 cup per serving

PREPARATION TIME
5 minutes

COOKING TIME
18 to 20 minutes

PER SERVING
Calories 155
Total Fat 3.0 g
  Saturated Fat 0.0 g
  Trans Fat 0.0 g
  Polyunsaturated Fat 1.0 g
  Monounsaturated Fat 1.5 g
Cholesterol 0 mg
Sodium 56 mg
Carbohydrates 28 g
  Fiber 6 g
  Sugars 4 g
Protein 5 g
Dietary Exchanges
  1½ starch, 1 vegetable,
  ½ fat

This peppery pasta side dish lends itself well to just about any vegetable combo you can imagine. Try it with your family's favorites or use up the dribs and drabs you have in the freezer.

8	cups water
16	ounces frozen vegetables, any combination
4	ounces dried whole-grain fettuccine or linguine, broken into pieces
1	tablespoon light tub margarine
1	teaspoon sesame seeds, dry-roasted if desired
½	teaspoon toasted sesame oil
⅛ to ¼	teaspoon crushed red pepper flakes

In a large saucepan, bring the water to a boil, covered, over high heat. Stir in the vegetables and pasta. Return to a boil. Reduce the heat and boil gently, uncovered, for 8 minutes, or until the pasta is tender and the vegetables are tender-crisp. Drain well in a colander. Pour into a serving bowl.

Add the remaining ingredients, stirring to coat.

sugar-kissed snow peas and carrots

SERVES 4
½ cup per serving

PREPARATION TIME
5 minutes

COOKING TIME
15 minutes

PER SERVING
Calories 48
Total Fat 1.5 g
  Saturated Fat 0.0 g
  Trans Fat 0.0 g
  Polyunsaturated Fat 0.5 g
  Monounsaturated Fat 0.5 g
Cholesterol 0 mg
Sodium 44 mg
Carbohydrates 8 g
  Fiber 2 g
  Sugars 5 g
Protein 1 g
Dietary Exchanges
  1 vegetable, ½ fat

The natural sweetness of peas and carrots is accented with just a bit of sugar.

1 cup water
8 ounces baby carrots
4 ounces snow peas, trimmed
1 tablespoon light tub margarine
1 teaspoon sugar

In a large saucepan, bring the water to a boil over high heat. Add the carrots. Return to a boil. Reduce the heat and simmer, covered, for 5 minutes.

Stir in the snow peas. Increase the heat to high and return to a boil. Reduce the heat and simmer, covered, for 3 minutes, or until the carrots and snow peas are tender-crisp. Drain well in a colander.

In the same pan, cook the margarine and sugar over medium heat until the margarine is melted, stirring once or twice. Stir in the vegetables. Cook for 2 minutes, or until the vegetables are glazed, stirring occasionally to coat.

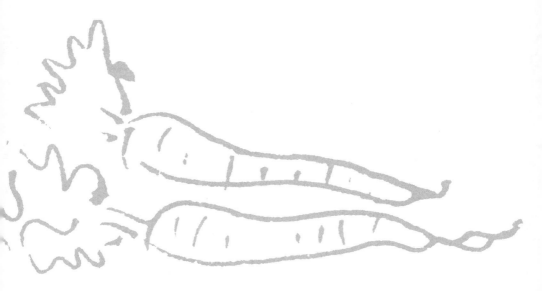

fresh herb polenta

SERVES 6
½ cup per serving

PREPARATION TIME
7 minutes

COOKING TIME
7 to 8 minutes

CHILLING TIME
at least 1 hour (optional)

BAKING TIME
30 minutes (optional)

PER SERVING
Calories 69
Total Fat 1.0 g
  Saturated Fat 0.5 g
  Trans Fat 0.0 g
  Polyunsaturated Fat 0.0 g
  Monounsaturated Fat 0.5 g
Cholesterol 2 mg
Sodium 109 mg
Carbohydrates 13 g
  Fiber 1 g
  Sugars 0 g
Protein 3 g
Dietary Exchanges
  1 starch

Tired of the same-old, same-old mashed potatoes? Serve this creamy polenta instead. For soft polenta, cook the cornmeal mixture only on the stovetop. Add the baking and chilling steps for a firmer version.

- 2 **cups water and ⅔ cup water, divided use**
- ⅔ **cup finely ground yellow cornmeal**
- ⅛ **teaspoon salt**
- ¼ **cup shredded or grated Parmesan cheese**
- 2 **tablespoons snipped fresh basil or 1 teaspoon dried, crumbled**
- 1 **teaspoon snipped fresh thyme or ¼ teaspoon dried, crumbled**
  Cooking spray (if baking)

In a medium saucepan, bring 2 cups water to a boil over high heat.

Meanwhile, in a large liquid measuring cup (to make pouring easy), stir together the cornmeal, salt, and remaining ⅔ cup water. Very slowly pour the mixture into the boiling water, stirring constantly. Return to a boil. Reduce the heat to low and cook for 5 minutes, or until the polenta is thick and pulls away from the side of the pan, stirring constantly. Stir in the Parmesan, basil, and thyme. To serve soft polenta, spoon onto plates.

For firmer polenta, continue by lightly spraying a 9-inch pie pan with cooking spray. Pour the hot polenta into the pie pan. Cover and refrigerate for at least 1 hour, or until firm (can be chilled overnight).

About 40 minutes before serving, preheat the oven to 350°F.

Bake the polenta for 30 minutes, or until heated through.

crisp skin-on oven fries

SERVES 4
6 potato wedges
per serving

PREPARATION TIME
8 minutes

COOKING TIME
20 minutes

PER SERVING
Calories 127
Total Fat 0.0 g
 Saturated Fat 0.0 g
 Trans Fat 0.0 g
 Polyunsaturated Fat 0.0 g
 Monounsaturated Fat 0.0 g
Cholesterol 0 mg
Sodium 154 mg
Carbohydrates 29 g
 Fiber 2 g
 Sugars 1 g
Protein 4 g
Dietary Exchanges
 2 starch

Keep the skin on these faux fries for all the nutrients—and crispness—they provide.

    Cooking spray
¼ teaspoon salt
¼ teaspoon paprika
¼ teaspoon garlic powder
⅛ teaspoon pepper
3 medium baking potatoes, each cut into 8 wedges

Preheat the oven to 450°F. Lightly spray a large baking sheet with cooking spray.

In a small bowl, stir together the salt, paprika, garlic powder, and pepper.

Arrange the potatoes with the skin side down in a single layer on the baking sheet. Lightly spray the potatoes with cooking spray. Sprinkle with the salt mixture.

Bake for 20 minutes, or until the potatoes are tender and the skins are crisp.

garlic quinoa

SERVES 4
¾ cup per serving

PREPARATION TIME
4 minutes

COOKING TIME
20 minutes

PER SERVING
Calories 167
Total Fat 2.5 g
 Saturated Fat 0.5 g
 Trans Fat 0.0 g
 Polyunsaturated Fat 1.5 g
 Monounsaturated Fat 0.5 g
Cholesterol 0 mg
Sodium 152 mg
Carbohydrates 30 g
 Fiber 3 g
 Sugars 1 g
Protein 6 g
Dietary Exchanges
 2 starch

Serve this high-protein, garlic-infused side dish as part of a vegetarian dinner or with a saucy main dish, such as Chicken with Leeks and Tomatoes (page 111).

    Cooking spray
½ cup chopped onion
2 teaspoons bottled minced garlic or 4 medium garlic cloves, minced
2 cups water
1 cup uncooked prerinsed quinoa
¼ teaspoon salt

Lightly spray a medium saucepan with cooking spray. Cook the onion and garlic over medium heat for 3 minutes, stirring frequently.

Stir in the water, quinoa, and salt. Increase the heat to high and bring to a boil. Reduce the heat and simmer, covered, for 15 minutes, or until the water is absorbed.

brown rice pilaf
WITH MUSHROOMS

SERVES 6
½ cup per serving

PREPARATION TIME
10 minutes

COOKING TIME
18 minutes

PER SERVING
Calories 108
Total Fat 1.0 g
  Saturated Fat 0.0 g
  Trans Fat 0.0 g
  Polyunsaturated Fat 0.5 g
  Monounsaturated Fat 0.5 g
Cholesterol 0 mg
Sodium 112 mg
Carbohydrates 21 g
  Fiber 3 g
  Sugars 2 g
Protein 3 g
Dietary Exchanges
  1½ starch

Try this speedy side dish with Steak with Sun-Dried Tomatoes (page 147) and your favorite green vegetable.

Cooking spray
8 ounces presliced button mushrooms (about 2½ cups)
6 to 8 medium green onions, sliced
1 teaspoon bottled minced garlic or 2 medium garlic cloves, minced
1¼ cups water
1 teaspoon very low sodium beef bouillon granules
¼ teaspoon salt
¼ teaspoon dried thyme, crumbled
1½ cups uncooked instant brown rice
¼ cup snipped fresh parsley (optional)

Lightly spray a medium saucepan with cooking spray. Cook the mushrooms, green onions, and garlic over medium-high heat for 5 minutes, or until the mushrooms are soft, stirring occasionally.

Stir in the water, bouillon granules, salt, and thyme. Increase the heat to high and bring to a boil. Stir in the rice. Return to a boil. Reduce the heat and simmer, covered, for 10 minutes, or until the rice is tender. Stir in the parsley.

southwestern rice

SERVES 4
¾ cup per serving

PREPARATION TIME
5 to 6 minutes

COOKING TIME
50 to 55 minutes

PER SERVING
Calories 169
Total Fat 1.5 g
  Saturated Fat 0.5 g
  Trans Fat 0.0 g
  Polyunsaturated Fat 0.5 g
  Monounsaturated Fat 0.5 g
Cholesterol 0 mg
Sodium 114 mg
Carbohydrates 35 g
  Fiber 2 g
  Sugars 1 g
Protein 5 g
Dietary Exchanges
  2½ starch

Fresh, nutty, and tangy are just a few of the words you'll think of when you taste this wonderfully flavorful rice dish.

2½ cups fat-free, low-sodium chicken broth
 ⅛ teaspoon salt
  1 cup uncooked brown aromatic rice, such as brown basmati or brown Texmati
 ½ teaspoon ground cumin
  1 medium tomatillo or tomato, chopped
  1 to 2 tablespoons snipped fresh cilantro
 ½ teaspoon grated lime zest
  1 teaspoon fresh lime juice
 ½ teaspoon minced fresh jalapeño

In a medium saucepan, bring the broth and salt to a boil over high heat. Stir in the rice and cumin. Return to a boil. Reduce the heat and simmer, covered, for 45 to 50 minutes, or until the rice is tender and the liquid is absorbed.

Stir in the remaining ingredients.

COOK'S TIP ON TOMATILLOS
Tomatillos (tohm-ah-TEE-ohs), also called Mexican green tomatoes, are small green fruits encased in thin, papery husks; they have a slightly acidic flavor with hints of lemon. Choose hard-fleshed tomatillos, discard the husks just before use, and wash the tomatillos well. To store them, leave the husks on and refrigerate the tomatillos in a paper bag for two to four weeks.

spanish spinach

SERVES 4
½ cup per serving

PREPARATION TIME
8 to 10 minutes

COOKING TIME
13 to 15 minutes

PER SERVING

Calories 53
Total Fat 2.5 g
  Saturated Fat 0.5 g
  Trans Fat 0.0 g
  Polyunsaturated Fat 0.5 g
  Monounsaturated Fat 1.5 g
Cholesterol 0 mg
Sodium 131 mg
Carbohydrates 6 g
  Fiber 2 g
  Sugars 3 g
Protein 3 g
Dietary Exchanges
  1 vegetable, ½ fat

"Spanish Spinach"—fun to say and good to eat! Serve this side dish with Salmon and Brown Rice Bake (page 82) or Baked Dijon Chicken (page 116).

2	teaspoons olive oil
1	small onion, thinly sliced
½	teaspoon bottled minced garlic or 1 medium garlic clove, minced
½	teaspoon paprika, smoked paprika, or hot paprika
½	teaspoon ground cumin
⅛	teaspoon salt
	Pinch of crushed red pepper flakes
10	ounces spinach (about 10 cups)
2	tablespoons water
1	medium Italian plum (Roma) tomato, chopped
2	teaspoons red wine vinegar

In a large nonstick skillet, heat the oil over medium heat, swirling to coat the bottom. Cook the onion for 5 minutes, or until softened and lightly browned, stirring frequently.

Stir in the garlic, paprika, cumin, salt, and red pepper flakes. Cook for 1 minute, stirring constantly.

Increase the heat to medium high. Stir in half the spinach and 1 tablespoon water. Cook for 2 to 3 minutes, or until the spinach is wilted, tossing constantly with tongs. Repeat.

Stir in the tomato. Cook for 1 minute, or just until heated through. Remove from the heat.

Stir in the vinegar.

COOK'S TIP
Buy a 10-ounce package of prewashed spinach so you won't need to rinse out the sand from the spinach.

summer-squash cakes

SERVES 4
1 cake per serving

PREPARATION TIME
10 minutes

COOKING TIME
12 to 15 minutes

PER SERVING
Calories 79
Total Fat 5.0 g
  Saturated Fat 1.5 g
  Trans Fat 0.0 g
  Polyunsaturated Fat 0.5 g
  Monounsaturated Fat 2.5 g
Cholesterol 57 mg
Sodium 108 mg
Carbohydrates 4 g
  Fiber 1 g
  Sugars 3 g
Protein 5 g
Dietary Exchanges
  1 vegetable, 1 fat

Lighten up traditional potato cakes by substituting zucchini and yellow summer squash. Sprinkling Parmesan on top gives you more flavor than stirring it into the cakes.

1 **large egg**
2 **tablespoons finely chopped shallot**
½ **teaspoon dried Italian seasoning, crumbled**
¼ **teaspoon pepper**
1 **cup shredded zucchini (about 1 medium)**
1 **cup shredded yellow summer squash (about 1 medium)**
2 **teaspoons olive oil**
¼ **cup shredded or grated Parmesan cheese**

In a medium bowl, using a fork, lightly beat the egg. Stir in the shallot, Italian seasoning, and pepper. Stir in the squashes.

In a large nonstick skillet, heat the oil over medium heat, swirling to coat the bottom. When the oil is hot, scoop the squash mixture by packed, heaping ⅓-cup portions (you will have 4 of these) into the skillet. Using the bottom of the measuring cup, gently press each cake to 3½ inches in diameter. Cook for 5 to 6 minutes on each side, or until crisp and golden, pressing again after turning. Just before serving, sprinkle with the Parmesan.

COOK'S TIP
To make Summer-Squash Cake appetizers, follow the cooking procedure above but spoon 28 to 30 heaping teaspoons of the squash mixture into the hot skillet (no need to press) and reduce the cooking time to 2 to 3 minutes on each side.

italian-style spaghetti squash

SERVES 6
½ cup per serving

PREPARATION TIME
5 minutes

MICROWAVE TIME
10 to 14 minutes

PER SERVING
Calories 56
Total Fat 1.0 g
  Saturated Fat 0.5 g
  Trans Fat 0.0 g
  Polyunsaturated Fat 0.0 g
  Monounsaturated Fat 0.5 g
Cholesterol 2 mg
Sodium 82 mg
Carbohydrates 10 g
  Fiber 2 g
  Sugars 5 g
Protein 2 g
Dietary Exchanges
  ½ starch

When you want a vegetable to serve with dinner but are thinking pasta, this dish will fill the bill.

- ½ **medium spaghetti squash (about 1½ pounds), seeds and strings discarded**
- 2 **tablespoons water**
- 1 **14.5-ounce can no-salt-added stewed tomatoes, drained**
- ¼ **teaspoon dried Italian seasoning, crumbled**
- ⅛ **teaspoon pepper**
- ¼ **cup shredded or grated Parmesan cheese**

Put the squash with the cut side down in a microwaveable baking dish. Add the water. Microwave, covered, on 100 percent power (high) for 10 to 14 minutes, or until the pulp can just be pierced with a fork. Drain well.

Using a potholder, hold the squash in one hand. With a fork, shred the pulp into strands, letting them fall into the baking dish.

Stir in the tomatoes, Italian seasoning, and pepper. Sprinkle with the Parmesan.

COOK'S TIP
Buy a 3-pound squash and cut it in half lengthwise. Use one piece for this recipe, and cover and refrigerate the other piece to use later. The uncooked squash will stay fresh for up to one week. Use it as you would spaghetti, such as with either pasta sauce or fresh herbs and olive oil, or toss the cooked squash with vinaigrette and vegetables, then chill the mixture and serve it like a pasta salad.

savory sweet potato sauté

SERVES 4
½ cup per serving

PREPARATION TIME
8 minutes

COOKING TIME
15 minutes

PER SERVING
Calories 139
Total Fat 4.5 g
  Saturated Fat 0.5 g
  Trans Fat 0.0 g
  Polyunsaturated Fat 0.5 g
  Monounsaturated Fat 3.5 g
Cholesterol 0 mg
Sodium 122 mg
Carbohydrates 23 g
  Fiber 4 g
  Sugars 6 g
Protein 2 g
Dietary Exchanges
  1 starch, 1 vegetable, 1 fat

A hint of thyme gives that savory touch to these shredded sweet potatoes. Break out of the mold and serve them instead of the expected mashed potatoes with Quick-Fix Chicken-Fried Steak (page 152), or give them a try with Lemony Chicken with Tarragon Oil (page 109).

1 teaspoon olive oil and 1 tablespoon olive oil, divided use

1½ cups diced onions

1 teaspoon bottled minced garlic or 2 medium garlic cloves, minced

1½ teaspoons finely chopped fresh thyme or ½ teaspoon dried, crumbled

2 small sweet potatoes (about 6 ounces each), peeled and shredded (coarsely shredded preferred)

⅛ teaspoon salt

In a large nonstick skillet, heat 1 teaspoon oil over medium-high heat, swirling to coat the bottom. Cook the onions for 3 minutes, or until soft, stirring frequently.

Stir in the garlic, thyme, and remaining 1 tablespoon oil. Cook for 15 seconds, stirring constantly. Spread the mixture evenly. Sprinkle the sweet potatoes so they cover the bottom of the skillet. Reduce the heat to medium low. Cook for 5 minutes without stirring. Stir the mixture, scraping the bottom and side of the skillet.

Cook for 5 minutes, or until the sweet potatoes are just tender. Remove from the heat. Sprinkle with the salt.

roasted cajun-style veggies

SERVES 4
¾ cup per serving

PREPARATION TIME
15 minutes

COOKING TIME
15 minutes

STANDING TIME
5 minutes

PER SERVING

Calories 116
Total Fat 4.0 g
  Saturated Fat 0.5 g
  Trans Fat 0.0 g
  Polyunsaturated Fat 0.5 g
  Monounsaturated Fat 2.5 g
Cholesterol 0 mg
Sodium 110 mg
Carbohydrates 20 g
  Fiber 5 g
  Sugars 6 g
Protein 3 g
Dietary Exchanges
  ½ starch, 2 vegetable, 1 fat

A revamp of traditional roasted veggies, this dish gets a decidedly Cajun flavor from the corn, okra, tomatoes, and thyme.

Cooking spray
1 cup frozen whole-kernel corn, thawed and patted dry
4 ounces okra, trimmed, cut into ½-inch rounds
4 ounces green beans, trimmed, cut into 2-inch pieces
2 medium carrots, cut crosswise into ⅛-inch slices
1 cup grape tomatoes
2 tablespoons snipped fresh parsley
1 tablespoon olive oil (extra-virgin preferred)
1½ teaspoons snipped fresh thyme or ½ teaspoon dried, crumbled
⅛ teaspoon salt

Preheat the oven to 425°F. Line a large baking sheet with aluminum foil. Lightly spray the foil with cooking spray.

Spread the corn, okra, beans, carrots, and tomatoes in a single layer on the baking sheet.

Roast for 10 minutes. Stir. Roast for 5 minutes, or until the carrots are tender. Remove from the oven.

With the vegetables still on the baking sheet, fold the edges of the foil to the center. Fold together to seal tightly. Let stand for 5 minutes so the flavors blend and the vegetables release some of their juices.

Transfer the vegetables and any accumulated juices to a medium bowl. Add the remaining ingredients, tossing gently to combine.

breads and breakfast dishes

easy mexican cornbread

Whip up a batch of this flavorful cornbread to serve with Hearty Pork and Onion Stew (page 159) or Three-Bean Chili (page 182).

> Cooking spray
> 1½ cups yellow cornmeal
> ½ cup whole-wheat flour
> ¼ cup sugar
> ½ teaspoon baking soda
> ½ teaspoon chili powder
> ½ teaspoon ground cumin
> ½ teaspoon cayenne
> 1½ cups low-fat buttermilk
> 1 11-ounce can whole-kernel corn with red and green bell peppers, drained
> 1 small red bell pepper, finely chopped
> 1 small fresh jalapeño, minced
> ⅓ cup canola or corn oil
> 2 large egg whites, lightly beaten with a fork

Preheat the oven to 425°F. Lightly spray a 13 × 9 × 2-inch baking pan with cooking spray. Set aside.

In a large bowl, stir together the cornmeal, flour, sugar, baking soda, chili powder, cumin, and cayenne.

In a medium bowl, stir together the remaining ingredients. Add to the cornmeal mixture, stirring until well combined. Pour into the baking pan, lightly smoothing the top.

Bake for 15 minutes, or until a wooden toothpick inserted near the center comes out clean and the top is golden brown. Transfer to a cooling rack and let cool for 5 minutes before slicing.

garden herb biscuits

SERVES 12
1 biscuit per serving

PREPARATION TIME
10 minutes

BAKING TIME
8 to 10 minutes

PER SERVING
Calories 76
Total Fat 1.0 g
 Saturated Fat 0.0 g
 Trans Fat 0.0 g
 Polyunsaturated Fat 0.0 g
 Monounsaturated Fat 0.5 g
Cholesterol 0 mg
Sodium 131 mg
Carbohydrates 15 g
 Fiber 1 g
 Sugars 2 g
Protein 2 g
Dietary Exchanges
 1 starch

You'll find tasty bits of green onions, carrot, and dillweed in each tender biscuit. Replace the dillweed with a different herb, such as marjoram, basil, or rosemary, for an easy variation.

   Cooking spray
1 cup reduced-fat baking and pancake mix and 2 tablespoons reduced-fat baking and pancake mix (lowest sodium available), divided use
¾ cup all-purpose flour
2 medium green onions, finely chopped
1 small carrot, grated
¼ teaspoon dried dillweed, crumbled
¾ cup fat-free milk

Preheat the oven to 450°F. Lightly spray a baking sheet with cooking spray. Set aside.

In a medium bowl, stir together 1 cup baking mix, the flour, green onions, carrot, and dillweed. Pour in the milk, stirring just until a soft dough forms. If the dough is sticky, gradually stir in enough of the remaining 2 tablespoons baking mix to make the dough easier to handle.

Drop the dough by tablespoonfuls onto the baking sheet (you should have 12 biscuits).

Bake for 8 to 10 minutes, or until the biscuits are lightly browned on top. Transfer the biscuits from the baking sheet to a cooling rack.

COOK'S TIP
You can freeze any leftover biscuits, then thaw them and heat on a baking sheet in a preheated 350°F oven for 3 to 5 minutes.

bran muffin breakfast trifle

SERVES 6
1 cup per serving

PREPARATION TIME
10 minutes

CHILLING TIME
at least 6 hours

PER SERVING
Calories 177
Total Fat 1.5 g
  Saturated Fat 0.0 g
  Trans Fat 0.0 g
  Polyunsaturated Fat 0.5 g
  Monounsaturated Fat 0.5 g
Cholesterol 2 mg
Sodium 127 mg
Carbohydrates 37 g
  Fiber 3 g
  Sugars 28 g
Protein 7 g
Dietary Exchanges
  1 starch, 1 fruit,
  ½ fat-free milk

As you'll discover with this dish, trifle doesn't have to be calorie-laden and it doesn't have to be served as dessert. Since you can make it the day before you need it, this mouthwatering version is terrific for a speedy, nutritious breakfast. With lots of fresh fruit to add appealing color, the trifle would be perfect as the centerpiece for your next brunch. Just be sure to save three bran muffins from Refrigerator Bran Muffins (page 234) to make it.

3 **bran muffins from Refrigerator Bran Muffins, coarsely crumbled (about 3 cups)**
3½ **cups assorted fruit and ½ cup assorted fruit, such as peeled kiwifruit, cantaloupe cubes, hulled strawberries, blueberries, blackberries, raspberries, and chopped mangoes, or any combination, divided use**
2 **cups fat-free vanilla or fruit-flavored yogurt**

In a 2½-quart glass bowl, such as a trifle bowl, or airtight container, layer as follows: half the muffin crumbs, 3½ cups fruit, the remaining muffin crumbs, the yogurt, and the remaining ½ cup fruit. Cover and refrigerate for at least 6 hours.

refrigerator bran muffins

SERVES 15
1 muffin per serving

PREPARATION TIME
12 to 15 minutes

BAKING TIME
15 to 18 minutes

OR

MICROWAVE TIME
30 to 50 seconds
(for one muffin)

STANDING TIME
5 minutes

PER SERVING
Calories 108
Total Fat 2.0 g
 Saturated Fat 0.0 g
 Trans Fat 0.0 g
 Polyunsaturated Fat 0.5 g
 Monounsaturated Fat 1.0 g
Cholesterol 0 mg
Sodium 131 mg
Carbohydrates 20 g
 Fiber 2 g
 Sugars 9 g
Protein 3 g
Dietary Exchanges
 1½ starch

Keep this muffin batter in the refrigerator for up to one week, baking as many muffins at a time as you need. Be sure to save three of them so you can make Bran Muffin Breakfast Trifle (page 233).

Cooking spray (optional)
 1 cup all-purpose flour
 ¾ cup unprocessed wheat bran
 ½ cup whole-wheat flour
 2½ teaspoons baking powder
 1 teaspoon ground cinnamon
 ¼ teaspoon salt
 1 cup fat-free milk
 ½ cup egg substitute
 ⅓ cup firmly packed light brown sugar
 ¼ cup unsweetened applesauce
 2 tablespoons canola or corn oil
 ⅓ cup raisins, chopped dates, or mixed dried
  fruit bits

If baking the muffins right after preparing the batter, preheat the oven to 400°F. If baking all 15 muffins, lightly spray one 12-cup muffin pan and 3 cups of a second muffin pan with cooking spray or use paper bake cups.

In a large bowl, stir together the all-purpose flour, wheat bran, whole-wheat flour, baking powder, cinnamon, and salt. Make a well in the center.

In a medium bowl, stir together the milk, egg substitute, brown sugar, applesauce, and oil. Add to the well in the flour mixture, stirring until the batter is just moistened but no flour is visible. Don't overmix; the batter should be thick and lumpy. Fold in the raisins. Use the batter immediately or transfer to an airtight container and refrigerate for up to one week.

Whether you are baking the muffins right away or refrigerating the batter, don't stir the batter again. Fill the desired number of muffin cups two-thirds full with batter. Fill the empty cups with water so the muffins bake evenly and the pan doesn't warp.

Bake for 15 to 18 minutes, or until the muffins are browned.

MICROWAVE METHOD

Combine the ingredients as directed. Line one or two 6-ounce custard cups with paper bake cups. Spoon 3 tablespoons batter into each cup. For one muffin, microwave on 100 percent power (high) for 30 to 50 seconds, or until done. For two muffins, microwave for 50 seconds to 1 minute, or until done. Let stand for 5 minutes.

COOK'S TIP ON WHEAT BRAN

An excellent source of fiber, wheat bran—also known as miller's bran—is the outer layer of wheat berries. Among its many uses, wheat bran adds nutrients and texture to baked goods, coatings, and meat loaf or hamburgers.

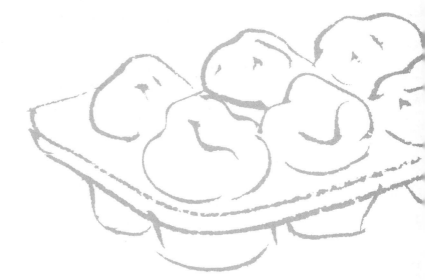

apple-spice coffee cake
WITH WALNUTS

SERVES 10
1 wedge per serving

PREPARATION TIME
10 minutes

COOKING TIME
31 to 36 minutes

COOLING TIME
1 hour 10 minutes

PER SERVING
Calories 177
Total Fat 5.0 g
  Saturated Fat 0.5 g
  Trans Fat 0.0 g
  Polyunsaturated Fat 2.0 g
  Monounsaturated Fat 2.5 g
Cholesterol 22 mg
Sodium 133 mg
Carbohydrates 30 g
  Fiber 2 g
  Sugars 18 g
Protein 4 g
Dietary Exchanges
  2 other carbohydrate, 1 fat

Shredded apple helps make this coffee cake moist, and sliced apple on top makes a pretty and delicious garnish that's baked right into the cake.

Cooking spray
1 teaspoon canola or corn oil and 2 tablespoons canola or corn oil, divided use
1 medium Granny Smith apple, peeled and thinly sliced, and 1 medium Granny Smith apple, peeled and coarsely shredded, divided use
¾ cup whole-wheat flour
½ cup all-purpose flour
¼ cup sugar
2 teaspoons ground ginger
1 teaspoon baking powder
1 teaspoon ground cinnamon
¼ teaspoon baking soda
¼ teaspoon ground cloves
⅛ teaspoon salt
¾ cup low-fat buttermilk
⅓ cup light or dark molasses
1 large egg
½ teaspoon vanilla extract
2 tablespoons finely chopped walnuts

Preheat the oven to 350°F. Lightly spray an 8-inch round cake pan with cooking spray. Set aside.

In a large nonstick skillet, heat 1 teaspoon oil over medium-high heat, swirling to coat the bottom. Cook the apple slices for 5 minutes, or until soft and lightly browned, gently stirring occasionally. Transfer to a small plate. Set aside.

Meanwhile, in a large bowl, stir together the flours, sugar, ginger, baking powder, cinnamon, baking soda, cloves, and salt. Set aside.

In a medium bowl, whisk together the buttermilk, molasses, egg, vanilla, and remaining 2 tablespoons oil. Stir this mixture and the shredded apple into the flour mixture until the batter is just moistened but no flour is visible. Don't overmix. Pour into the pan, lightly smoothing the top.

Arrange the apple slices in an overlapping circle on the center of the batter. Sprinkle the walnuts over the batter.

Bake for 25 to 30 minutes, or until a wooden toothpick inserted in the center comes out clean. Transfer the pan to a cooling rack and let cool for 10 minutes. Place a large plate over the pan and flip the coffee cake onto the plate. Remove the pan. Immediately flip the cake back onto the cooling rack (the apple side will face up). Let stand for about 1 hour, or until completely cool.

confetti scrambler

SERVES 4
½ cup per serving

PREPARATION TIME
5 minutes

COOKING TIME
4 minutes

PER SERVING
Calories 72
Total Fat 2.0 g
  Saturated Fat 0.5 g
  Trans Fat 0.0 g
  Polyunsaturated Fat 0.0 g
  Monounsaturated Fat 1.0 g
Cholesterol 2 mg
Sodium 233 mg
Carbohydrates 3 g
  Fiber 1 g
  Sugars 2 g
Protein 10 g
Dietary Exchanges
  1½ very lean meat

Colorful, flavorful, versatile, and super fast to make, this dish is good with toast and fruit for breakfast, or try it for a quick lunch with a green salad and a whole-grain roll.

  1 **teaspoon olive oil**
1½ **cups egg substitute**
  2 **medium green onions, finely chopped**
 ¼ **cup finely chopped tomatoes**
  2 **tablespoons shredded or grated Parmesan cheese**

In a large nonstick skillet, heat the oil over medium heat, swirling to coat the bottom. Cook the egg substitute for 1 minute without stirring. Sprinkle with the green onions and tomatoes. Stir gently. Cook for 1 minute without stirring, or until the desired doneness. Remove from the heat.

    Sprinkle with the Parmesan. Serve immediately for peak flavor.

rise-and-shine cookies

SERVES 15
2 cookies per serving

PREPARATION TIME
10 minutes

BAKING TIME
10 minutes

PER SERVING
Calories 112
Total Fat 3.5 g
  Saturated Fat 0.5 g
  Trans Fat 0.0 g
  Polyunsaturated Fat 1.0 g
  Monounsaturated Fat 2.0 g
Cholesterol 0 mg
Sodium 92 mg
Carbohydrates 18 g
  Fiber 2 g
  Sugars 7 g
Protein 3 g
Dietary Exchanges
  1 starch, ½ fat

Cookies for breakfast? Sure—when they are rich in fiber and low in fat and taste like big chunks of granola!

½ cup all-purpose flour
¼ cup whole-wheat flour
½ teaspoon baking soda
¼ teaspoon salt
¼ teaspoon ground cinnamon
⅛ teaspoon ground nutmeg
½ cup firmly packed brown sugar
¼ cup egg substitute
3 tablespoons canola or corn oil
1¼ cups quick-cooking oatmeal or regular rolled oats
½ cup wheat germ

Preheat the oven to 350°F.

In a small bowl, stir together the flours, baking soda, salt, cinnamon, and nutmeg.

In a large bowl, stir together the brown sugar, egg substitute, and oil. Stir in the flour mixture, oatmeal, and wheat germ.

Drop the dough by tablespoons about 1 inch apart on the baking sheet. Using your hand or the bottom of a glass, flatten slightly to a 2-inch diameter.

Bake the cookies for 10 minutes, or until light brown. Transfer to cooling racks. Serve or let cool completely and store in an airtight container at room temperature for up to one week or freeze in a resealable plastic freezer bag for up to three weeks.

whole-wheat buttermilk pancakes
WITH BLUEBERRY-MAPLE SYRUP

SERVES 4
2 pancakes, heaping
1 tablespoon syrup,
and ¼ cup blueberries
per serving

PREPARATION TIME
10 minutes

COOKING TIME
5 to 12 minutes

PER SERVING
Calories 344
Total Fat 6.5 g
  Saturated Fat 1.0 g
  Trans Fat 0.0 g
  Polyunsaturated Fat 1.5 g
  Monounsaturated Fat 3.0 g
Cholesterol 56 mg
Sodium 453 mg
Carbohydrates 64 g
  Fiber 5 g
  Sugars 27 g
Protein 10 g
Dietary Exchanges
  3 starch, ½ fruit, 1 other
  carbohydrate, ½ fat

Start your day with a double dose of nutritious blueberries, one as part of the syrup and one to sprinkle over the pancakes.

PANCAKES
- 1 **cup whole-wheat flour**
- ½ **cup all-purpose flour**
- 2 **tablespoons sugar**
- 2 **teaspoons baking powder**
- ¼ **teaspoon baking soda**
- ⅛ **teaspoon salt**
- 1¼ **cups low-fat buttermilk**
- 1 **large egg**
- 1 **tablespoon canola or corn oil**
- 1 **teaspoon vanilla extract**

SYRUP
- ¼ **cup maple syrup**
- ¼ **cup blueberries**

- 1 **cup blueberries**

In a large bowl, stir together the flours, sugar, baking powder, baking soda, and salt.

In a small bowl, whisk together the remaining pancake ingredients. Pour into the flour mixture. Stir until the batter is just moistened but no flour is visible. Don't overmix; the batter should be slightly lumpy.

Preheat a nonstick griddle or large nonstick skillet over medium heat. Test the temperature by sprinkling a few drops of water on the griddle. If the water evaporates quickly, the griddle is ready.

Using a ¼-cup measure, pour the batter onto the griddle, spreading the batter into 3½-inch circles. (You may need to make two batches to get 8 pancakes.) Cook for 2 to 3 minutes, or until the tops are bubbly and the edges are dry. Turn over. Cook for 2 minutes, or until the bottoms are browned. Transfer to a warm plate and cover to keep warm. Repeat with any remaining batter.

Meanwhile, in a small saucepan, bring the maple syrup and ¼ cup blueberries to a boil over medium heat. Boil for 1 to 2 minutes, or until some of the blueberries pop.

Pour the syrup over the pancakes. Sprinkle with the remaining 1 cup blueberries.

COOK'S TIP
You can make the syrup using ¼ cup chopped hulled strawberries or ¼ cup raspberries instead of the ¼ cup blueberries. Sprinkle with the 1 cup blueberries if you wish.

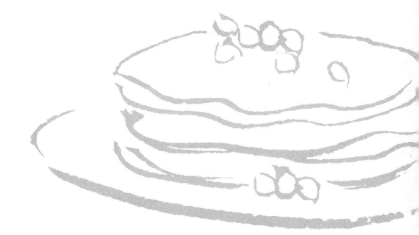

homemade muesli

SERVES 9
½ cup per serving

PREPARATION TIME
5 minutes

COOKING TIME
3 to 4 minutes

STANDING TIME
5 minutes

PER SERVING
Calories 173
Total Fat 3.0 g
  Saturated Fat 0.5 g
  Trans Fat 0.0 g
  Polyunsaturated Fat 1.0 g
  Monounsaturated Fat 1.5 g
Cholesterol 2 mg
Sodium 53 mg
Carbohydrates 33 g
  Fiber 3 g
  Sugars 21 g
Protein 6 g
Dietary Exchanges
  1 starch, 1 other
  carbohydrate, ½ fat

The beauty of this European-inspired cereal is that you combine all the dry ingredients for the entire batch, then make as many servings as you need each morning.

1   **cup uncooked rolled oats or quick-cooking oatmeal**
1   **cup whole-grain flakes or bran cereal**
1   **cup sweetened dried cranberries or mixed dried fruit bits**
⅓   **cup slivered almonds, dry-roasted**
¼   **cup firmly packed light brown sugar**
½   **teaspoon ground cinnamon**
3   **cups fat-free milk, divided use**

In a large bowl, stir together all the ingredients except the milk. Transfer to an airtight container.

For each serving, put ⅓ cup oat mixture in a cereal bowl. Stir in ⅓ cup milk. Let stand for 5 minutes so the oats soften.

overnight mixed-grain cereal

SERVES 14
²/₃ cup per serving

PREPARATION TIME
3 minutes

STANDING TIME
Overnight

COOKING TIME
6 to 11 minutes

PER SERVING
Calories 207
Total Fat 1.5 g
  Saturated Fat 0.0 g
  Trans Fat 0.0 g
  Polyunsaturated Fat 0.5 g
  Monounsaturated Fat 0.5 g
Cholesterol 0 mg
Sodium 2 mg
Carbohydrates 44 g
  Fiber 8 g
  Sugars 7 g
Protein 6 g
Dietary Exchanges
  3 starch

As you do with Homemade Muesli (page 242), combine the dry ingredients once, then cook only as many servings of cereal as you want. You do need to plan ahead so this cereal can soak in water overnight. The next morning, it will cook in just a few minutes. You may want to add a small amount of fat-free milk and a sprinkling of sugar to the cooked mixture.

1 **cup uncooked steel-cut oats**
1 **cup uncooked pearl barley**
1 **cup wheat berries**
1 **cup sweetened dried cranberries, dried
    blueberries, or chopped dates**
²/₃ **cup millet**

In a large airtight container, stir together all the ingredients.

For each serving, in a saucepan, stir together ⅓ cup cereal mixture and ⅔ cup water. Let stand, covered, at room temperature overnight.

In the morning, bring the cereal mixture to a boil, uncovered, over high heat. Reduce the heat and simmer for 5 to 10 minutes, stirring occasionally.

COOK'S TIP ON WHEAT BERRIES
Wheat berries are unprocessed whole kernels—both the bran and the germ—making them the most nutritious part of wheat. Also called groats, wheat berries have a robust, nutlike flavor and are brown and almost round. They need presoaking, or you will have to cook them for at least an hour to get them soft and chewy.

COOK'S TIP ON MILLET
Millet has been a staple in African and Asian cooking for thousands of years. It is a tiny pale yellow or reddish orange grain that contains no gluten. It has a delicate, bland flavor and, like couscous, cooks quickly and is fluffy.

mandarin breakfast parfaits

SERVES 4
²/₃ cup per serving

PREPARATION TIME
5 minutes

PER SERVING
Calories 184
Total Fat 1.5 g
  Saturated Fat 0.5 g
  Trans Fat 0.0 g
  Polyunsaturated Fat 0.5 g
  Monounsaturated Fat 0.5 g
Cholesterol 1 mg
Sodium 100 mg
Carbohydrates 39 g
  Fiber 2 g
  Sugars 29 g
Protein 7 g
Dietary Exchanges
  1 starch, 1 fruit,
  1 fat-free milk

No more excuses for not eating breakfast! All it takes is three ingredients and five minutes to have a colorful parfait that you can also use for a snack or even dessert. We like the mandarin oranges for a change from the more commonly used strawberries or bananas, but feel free to create your own combinations of fruits and yogurts for variety.

  2 11-ounce cans mandarin oranges, packed in water or light syrup, drained
 12 ounces fat-free vanilla or fruit-flavored yogurt
 ²/₃ cup low-fat granola without raisins

In parfait glasses, make a layer of half of each ingredient in the order listed. Repeat.

desserts

easy cherry-cinnamon crisp

SERVES 9
½ cup per serving

PREPARATION TIME
5 to 6 minutes

COOKING TIME
30 minutes

PER SERVING

Calories 96
Total Fat 2.5 g
    Saturated Fat 0.0 g
    Trans Fat 0.0 g
    Polyunsaturated Fat 0.5 g
    Monounsaturated Fat 1.0 g
Cholesterol 0 mg
Sodium 45 mg
Carbohydrates 17 g
    Fiber 1 g
    Sugars 9 g
Protein 2 g
Dietary Exchanges
    1 other carbohydrate, ½ fat

A crunchy oat-based topping adds a hint of sweetness to balance the tartness of the cherries in this homey dessert.

⅔ cup uncooked rolled oats
⅓ cup all-purpose flour
¼ cup firmly packed light brown sugar
1 teaspoon ground cinnamon
¼ cup light tub margarine
1 14.5-ounce can tart red cherries packed in water, drained

Preheat the oven to 375°F.

In a medium bowl, stir together the oats, flour, brown sugar, and cinnamon. Cut in the margarine until the mixture is crumbly.

Pour the cherries into an 8-inch square glass baking dish. Top with the oats mixture.

Bake for 30 minutes, or until the topping is light brown. Serve warm.

chocolate-banana mini cupcakes

SERVES 6
2 mini cupcakes
per serving

PREPARATION TIME
15 minutes

COOKING TIME
10 to 12 minutes

COOLING TIME
5 minutes

PER SERVING
Calories 114
Total Fat 4.0 g
  Saturated Fat 1.0 g
  Trans Fat 0.0 g
  Polyunsaturated Fat 1.0 g
  Monounsaturated Fat 2.0 g
Cholesterol 0 mg
Sodium 87 mg
Carbohydrates 19 g
  Fiber 1 g
  Sugars 10 g
Protein 2 g
Dietary Exchanges
  1½ other carbohydrate,
  1 fat

These mini cupcakes are a perfectly sized sweet treat to send in a lunch box or serve as an after-school snack.

   Cooking spray
¼ cup whole-wheat flour
¼ cup all-purpose flour
 3 tablespoons sugar
¼ teaspoon baking powder
⅛ teaspoon baking soda
   Pinch of salt
¼ cup mashed ripe banana (about ½ large)
¼ cup low-fat buttermilk
 1 tablespoon canola or corn oil
¼ teaspoon vanilla extract
 2 tablespoons mini chocolate chips or finely chopped semisweet chocolate
 1 large egg white

Preheat the oven to 400°F. Lightly spray a 12-cup mini muffin pan with cooking spray. Set aside.

In a medium bowl, whisk together the flours, sugar, baking powder, baking soda, and salt.

In a small bowl, whisk together the banana, buttermilk, oil, and vanilla. Stir into the flour mixture until the batter is just moistened but no flour is visible. Don't overmix; the batter should be slightly lumpy. Stir in the chocolate chips.

In a small mixing bowl, using an electric mixer on high speed, beat the egg white for 2 minutes, or until stiff peaks form (the peaks don't fall when the beaters are lifted). Using a rubber scraper, fold half the egg white at a time into the batter.

Spoon about 1 rounded tablespoonful of batter into each muffin cup.

Bake for 10 to 12 minutes, or until a wooden toothpick inserted into the center of a cupcake comes out clean. Transfer the pan to a cooling rack and let cool for 5 minutes. Serve the cupcakes warm or at room temperature.

cranberry-studded rice pudding
WITH SWEET ORANGE SAUCE

SERVES 6
½ cup pudding and
scant 1 tablespoon sauce
per serving

PREPARATION TIME
10 minutes (including for
sauce)

MICROWAVE TIME
2 to 3 minutes

COOKING TIME
55 minutes

STANDING TIME
15 minutes (optional)

CHILLING TIME
1 to 12 hours (optional)

PER SERVING
Calories 185
Total Fat 0.5 g
    Saturated Fat 0.0 g
    Trans Fat 0.0 g
    Polyunsaturated Fat 0.0 g
    Monounsaturated Fat 0.0 g
Cholesterol 0 mg
Sodium 124 mg
Carbohydrates 39 g
    Fiber 1 g
    Sugars 23 g
Protein 9 g
Dietary Exchanges
    2½ other carbohydrate,
    1 very lean meat

WITH SAUCE

Calories 224
Total Fat 1.0 g
    Saturated Fat 0.5 g
    Trans Fat 0.0 g
    Polyunsaturated Fat 0.5 g
    Monounsaturated Fat 0.5 g
Cholesterol 0 mg
Sodium 139 mg
Carbohydrates 47 g
    Fiber 1 g
    Sugars 29 g
Protein 9 g
Dietary Exchanges
    3 other carbohydrate,
    1 very lean meat

For this fruity rice pudding, all you need to do is warm the rice, combine the ingredients, and pop the pudding in the oven. You will have a delicious dessert even without the sauce, but with the sauce, it's super good! The pudding is equally tasty whether you serve it hot, at room temperature, or chilled, so you can prepare it at any time that's convenient for you.

Cooking spray
PUDDING
10 ounces frozen cooked brown rice (about 2 cups)
2 cups fat-free half-and-half
½ cup egg substitute
⅓ cup sugar
⅓ cup sweetened dried cranberries
1 teaspoon ground cinnamon
1 teaspoon vanilla extract

SAUCE (OPTIONAL)
2 tablespoons firmly packed dark brown sugar
⅔ cup fresh orange juice
2 teaspoons grated orange zest
1 tablespoon light tub margarine

Preheat the oven to 350°F. Lightly spray an 11 × 7 × 2-inch glass baking dish with cooking spray. Set aside.

Using the package directions, microwave the rice until warm. Transfer to a medium bowl. Stir in the remaining pudding ingredients. Pour into the baking dish.

Bake for 45 minutes. Stir. Bake for 10 minutes, or until the pudding has thickened (it won't be firm).

Meanwhile, to make the sauce, in a large saucepan, stir together the brown sugar and orange juice. Bring to a boil over high heat, stirring occasionally. Boil for 2 to 3 minutes, or until the mixture is reduced to ¼ cup, stirring occasionally. Remove from the heat.

Whisk in the orange zest and margarine. Set aside to cool slightly, until the pudding is done.

Spoon the pudding into custard cups or small ramekins. To serve the pudding hot, spoon the sauce over it. For room temperature, let the pudding stand for about 15 minutes, then spoon the sauce on top. To serve chilled, cover and refrigerate the pudding and sauce separately for 1 to 12 hours.

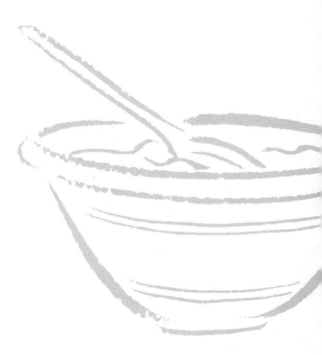

balsamic berries brûlée

SERVES 4
½ cup per serving

PREPARATION TIME
10 minutes

COOKING TIME
1 to 2 minutes

STANDING TIME
5 minutes

PER SERVING
Calories 96
Total Fat 0.0 g
　Saturated Fat 0.0 g
　Trans Fat 0.0 g
　Polyunsaturated Fat 0.0 g
　Monounsaturated Fat 0.0 g
Cholesterol 4 mg
Sodium 38 mg
Carbohydrates 21 g
　Fiber 2 g
　Sugars 16 g
Protein 3 g
Dietary Exchanges
　1½ other carbohydrate

You'll love how pepper and the tang of balsamic vinegar intensify the sweetness of fresh strawberries.

 2　**cups strawberries, hulled and thinly sliced**
 1　**teaspoon sugar**
 2　**tablespoons balsamic vinegar**
 1　**teaspoon chopped fresh mint**
 ⅛　**to ¼ teaspoon pepper, or to taste**
 ⅓　**cup fat-free sour cream**
 ⅓　**cup fat-free plain yogurt**
 2　**tablespoons firmly packed light brown sugar**

Preheat the broiler.

In a 9-inch pie pan, gently stir together the berries and sugar. Let stand for 5 minutes so the flavors blend.

Stir in the vinegar and mint. Sprinkle with the pepper.

In a small bowl, stir together the sour cream and yogurt. Spoon over the berry mixture. Sprinkle with the brown sugar.

Broil the berry mixture 4 to 6 inches from the heat for 1 to 2 minutes, or until the brown sugar melts. Serve immediately for peak texture and flavor.

COOK'S TIP
If you have a pepper mill, be sure to grind your own pepper for this recipe.

grilled peaches

WITH ALMOND LIQUEUR

SERVES 4
½ peach and ½ cup
frozen yogurt per serving

PREPARATION TIME
7 to 8 minutes

COOKING TIME
8 to 10 minutes

STANDING TIME
10 minutes

PER SERVING

Calories 170
Total Fat 1.5 g
  Saturated Fat 0.0 g
  Trans Fat 0.0 g
  Polyunsaturated Fat 0.5 g
  Monounsaturated Fat 1.0 g
Cholesterol 2 mg
Sodium 65 mg
Carbohydrates 32 g
  Fiber 2 g
  Sugars 29 g
Protein 6 g
Dietary Exchanges
  2 other carbohydrate, ½ fat

Grilled peaches with an almond-flavored glaze and a topping of frozen yogurt are a sweet ending for any outdoor barbecue.

    Cooking spray
2 teaspoons fresh lemon juice
1 teaspoon sugar
2 tablespoons almond-flavored liqueur
2 firm but ripe peaches, halved
2 cups fat-free vanilla frozen yogurt
½ teaspoon ground cinnamon
1 tablespoon plus 1 teaspoon slivered almonds, dry-roasted

Lightly spray the grill rack with cooking spray. Preheat the grill on medium high.

In a small bowl, stir together the lemon juice and sugar until the sugar is almost dissolved. Stir in the liqueur. Set aside.

Lightly spray the cut side of the peaches with cooking spray. Place the peaches with the cut side up on the grill. Grill for 3 minutes. Turn over. Grill for 2 to 3 minutes, or until heated through and slightly softened. Transfer the peaches with the cut side up to a small shallow baking dish.

Spoon the lemon juice mixture over the peaches. Let stand for 10 minutes, spooning the liquid over the peaches occasionally. Transfer the peaches with the cut side up to custard cups or small ramekins. Spoon any remaining liquid (there won't be much) into the peach cavities. Top with the frozen yogurt, cinnamon, and almonds.

COOK'S TIP

Look in the supermarket for unsalted almonds that have already been dry-roasted.

minty fruit parfaits

SERVES 4
heaping ½ cup
per serving

PREPARATION TIME
10 to 15 minutes

CHILLING TIME
15 to 30 minutes

PER SERVING
Calories 156
Total Fat 0.0 g
  Saturated Fat 0.0 g
  Trans Fat 0.0 g
  Polyunsaturated Fat 0.0 g
  Monounsaturated Fat 0.0 g
Cholesterol 10 mg
Sodium 75 mg
Carbohydrates 32 g
  Fiber 2 g
  Sugars 24 g
Protein 6 g
Dietary Exchanges
  1 fruit, 1 fat-free milk

Choose a variety of festive fruits, such as assorted berries, kiwifruit, grapes, and peaches, when making these cool, refreshing parfaits. Don't leave out the fresh mint; even though you use only a very small amount, it makes a deliciously big impact.

8   ounces fat-free sour cream
¼   cup confectioners' sugar
1   tablespoon chopped fresh mint
2   cups assorted cut fresh fruit
6   ounces fat-free lemon yogurt, lightly beaten with a fork if thick
4   sprigs of fresh mint (optional)

In a small bowl, stir together the sour cream, confectioners' sugar, and chopped mint. Spoon half into custard cups or small ramekins. Arrange half the fruit on top. Repeat. Refrigerate for at least 15 minutes (30 if possible). Just before serving, drizzle the yogurt over the fruit. Garnish with the mint sprigs.

COOK'S TIP
You can make the parfaits up to three days in advance. Cover them before refrigerating, and follow the directions above for adding the yogurt and mint.

sherbet parfaits

SERVES 4
1 parfait per serving

PREPARATION TIME
8 minutes

PER SERVING
Calories 164
Total Fat 0.0 g
  Saturated Fat 0.0 g
  Trans Fat 0.0 g
  Polyunsaturated Fat 0.0 g
  Monounsaturated Fat 0.0 g
Cholesterol 0 mg
Sodium 36 mg
Carbohydrates 39 g
  Fiber 4 g
  Sugars 27 g
Protein 1 g
Dietary Exchanges
  2½ other carbohydrate

Any sherbet will go nicely with the sweetened fruit, but rainbow sherbet looks especially pretty.

2 **cups raspberries or blueberries**
1 **tablespoon sugar**
1 **pint frozen sherbet, any flavor**

In a medium bowl, stir together the berries and sugar. Using a potato masher or fork, mash the berries slightly.

Spoon half the berries into parfait glasses. Spoon half the sherbet over the berries. Repeat. Serve immediately or freeze until serving time. If frozen, let stand at room temperature for 10 minutes before serving.

ice cream

WITH FRESH STRAWBERRY SAUCE

SERVES 4
½ cup ice cream and
heaping ¼ cup sauce
per serving

PREPARATION TIME
8 to 10 minutes

PER SERVING
Calories 137
Total Fat 0.0 g
  Saturated Fat 0.0 g
  Trans Fat 0.0 g
  Polyunsaturated Fat 0.0 g
  Monounsaturated Fat 0.0 g
Cholesterol 0 mg
Sodium 66 mg
Carbohydrates 31 g
  Fiber 1 g
  Sugars 21 g
Protein 4 g
Dietary Exchanges
  2 other carbohydrate

When fresh fruit is at its luscious best, drizzle this sauce over your favorite kind instead of over ice cream.

1 **cup strawberries, hulled**
1 **tablespoon sugar**
1 **tablespoon orange-flavored liqueur or fresh orange juice**
1 **pint fat-free ice cream, such as vanilla**

In a food processor or blender, process the strawberries, sugar, and liqueur until smooth.

Scoop the ice cream into bowls. Spoon the sauce (hot, warm, or chilled) on top. To make the sauce in advance, pour it into a small airtight container and refrigerate until serving time.

COOK'S TIP ON "FROSTY FRUIT"
Try making "Frosty Fruit," fresh fruit that is slightly frozen for a unique taste sensation, to serve as a dessert or to create a pretty garnish for cold fruit soups, summer salads, or other desserts. Use fruit such as grapes, whole small hulled strawberries, blueberries, raspberries, melon chunks, sliced peaches, or peeled kiwifruit chunks. Choose firm, ripe (but not overripe) fruit with no signs of bruises or blemishes. Rinse the fruit and pat dry. Arrange it in a single layer on a baking sheet. Freeze, uncovered, for 1 hour, or until firm. At serving time, remove from the freezer and let stand for 2 minutes.

dried-fruit truffles

SERVES 12
2 truffles per serving

PREPARATION TIME
10 minutes

PER SERVING
Calories 56
Total Fat 0.0 g
 Saturated Fat 0.0 g
 Trans Fat 0.0 g
 Polyunsaturated Fat 0.0 g
 Monounsaturated Fat 0.0 g
Cholesterol 0 mg
Sodium 1 mg
Carbohydrates 14 g
 Fiber 2 g
 Sugars 10 g
Protein 1 g
Dietary Exchanges
 1 fruit

No cooking is needed for this bite-size dessert, which has a surprising richness.

2 tablespoons unsweetened cocoa powder (dark preferred), sifted
Cooking spray
1 cup dried pitted plums (orange essence preferred)
½ cup dried pitted dates

Spread the cocoa powder in a medium shallow dish. Set aside.

Lightly spray the chopping blade of a food processor or blender with cooking spray. Process the dried plums and dates until finely chopped, scraping the side as necessary.

Moistening your hands periodically with cold water to keep the mixture from sticking, shape it into 24 truffles, each about 1 inch in diameter. After you make a truffle, transfer it to the dish. Turn the truffles to coat with cocoa powder. Transfer to a large piece of wax paper. Serve at room temperature. Refrigerate any leftover truffles in an airtight container for up to two weeks.

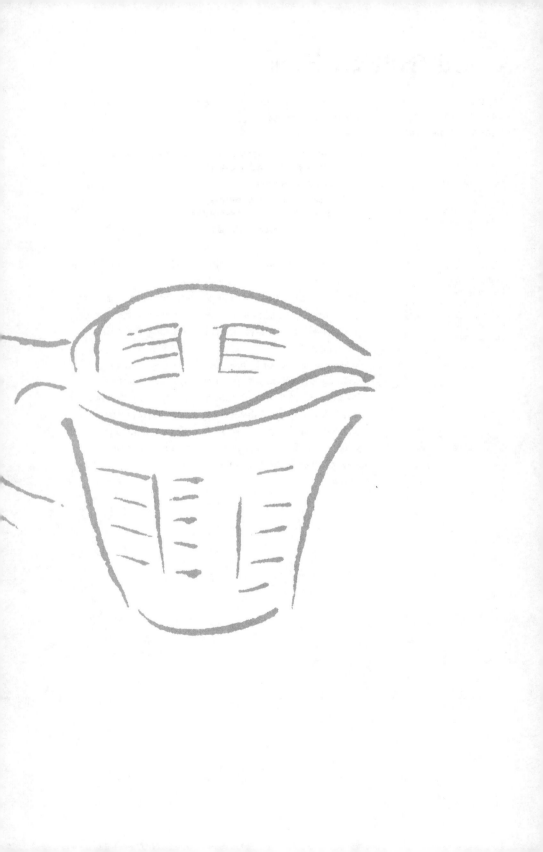

appendixes

APPENDIX A: **quick & easy weekly dinner planner**

	dinner menu plan	fresh/frozen ingredients	pantry staples
MON			
TUES			
WED			
THURS			
FRI			
SAT			
SUN			

APPENDIX B: **food groups and suggested servings**

For each basic food group, the following chart lists the average numbers of recommended servings, which are based on daily calorie intake. The number of servings that is right for you will vary depending on your caloric needs. When shopping, compare nutrition facts panels and look for the products that are lowest in sodium, saturated fat, trans fat, and cholesterol, and that don't have added sugars.

food group	calorie range			sample serving sizes
	1,600	**2,000**	**2,600**	
VEGETABLES Eat a variety of colors and types.	3 to 4 servings per day	4 to 5 servings per day	5 to 6 servings per day	1 cup raw leafy vegetable ½ cup cut-up raw or cooked nonleafy vegetable ½ cup vegetable juice
FRUITS Eat a variety of colors and types.	4 servings per day	4 to 5 servings per day	5 to 6 servings per day	1 medium fruit (about baseball size) ¼ cup dried fruit ½ cup fresh, frozen, or canned fruit ½ cup fruit juice
FIBER-RICH WHOLE GRAINS Choose whole grains for at least half of your servings.	6 servings per day	6 to 8 servings per day	10 to 11 servings per day	1 slice bread 1 oz dry cereal (check nutrition label for cup measurements) ½ cup cooked rice, pasta, or cereal
FAT-FREE, 1% FAT, AND LOW-FAT DAIRY PRODUCTS Choose fat-free when possible but compare sodium levels.	2 to 3 servings per day	2 to 3 servings per day	3 servings per day	1 cup milk 1 cup yogurt 1½ oz cheese
FISH Choose varieties rich in omega-3 fatty acids.	6 to 7 oz (cooked) per week	6 to 7 oz (cooked) per week	6 to 7 oz (cooked) per week	3 to 3½ oz cooked fish

chart continues ››

food group	calorie range			sample serving sizes
	1,600	2,000	2,600	
LEAN MEATS AND SKINLESS POULTRY Choose lean and extra-lean.	3 oz (cooked) per day	3 to 6 oz (cooked) per day	6 oz (cooked) per day	3 oz cooked meat or poultry
LEGUMES, NUTS, AND SEEDS Choose unsalted products.	3 servings per week	4 to 5 servings per week	1 serving per day	⅓ cup or 1½ oz nuts 2 Tb peanut butter 2 Tb or ½ oz seeds ½ cup cooked dried beans or peas
FATS AND OILS Use liquid vegetable oil and spray or light tub margarines most often. Choose products with the lowest amount of sodium.	2 servings per day	2 to 3 servings per day	2 to 3 servings per day	1 tsp light tub margarine 1 Tb light mayonnaise 1 tsp vegetable oil 1 Tb regular or 2 Tb light salad dressing (fat-free dressing does not count as a serving)

Adapted from the DASH (Dietary Approaches to Stop Hypertension) eating plan developed by the National Heart, Lung, and Blood Institute, National Institutes of Health.

APPENDIX C: **food safety tips**

Following a few easy tips will help keep your fresh and stored foods safe to eat. The basic steps in preventing the spread of bacteria as you prepare meals are:

- Clean: Wash your hands, kitchen surfaces, and cooking equipment often.
- Separate: Don't let raw foods contaminate others.
- Cook: Be sure cooked food reaches the proper temperature (see the first chart on page 262).
- Chill: Refrigerate or freeze foods promptly.

STORING FOODS BEFORE COOKING

As soon as you bring groceries home from the store, get them ready for safe storage. To store fresh vegetables and fruit, cut away any damaged or bruised areas and discard any produce that looks rotten. Just before eating, cutting, or cooking vegetables and fruits, wash them under running water and dry with a clean cloth towel or paper towel. (Washing fruits and vegetables with soap or detergent or using commercial produce washes is not recommended.)

Refrigerate meat and poultry as soon as possible to slow the growth of bacteria. These foods can be refrigerated or frozen in the original packaging if they will be used soon. If refrigerated, keep meat and poultry at 40°F or below and use within one or two days. To freeze a quantity of raw steaks or chicken breasts, discard all visible fat and stack the food in layers, separated by sheets of wax paper. Then place in airtight freezer bags or other freezer-proof containers.

MEAT	GROUND AND CUBED—3 to 4 months CHOPS—4 to 6 months STEAKS AND ROASTS—6 to 12 months
POULTRY	GROUND—3 to 4 months BREASTS AND PIECES—9 months WHOLE BIRD—1 year
FISH	FATTY FISH (salmon, tuna)—2 to 3 months SHELLFISH (shrimp, scallops, clams)—3 to 6 months LEAN FISH (tilapia, sole, cod)—6 months
BROTHS AND SOUPS	2 to 3 months
BERRIES	4 to 6 months
CHEESES	6 months
VEGETABLES	8 months
JUICES	8 to 12 months

Frozen foods kept at a consistent temperature of 0°F will stay safe to eat indefinitely, but keeping them longer than the time frames recommended will affect the quality of the food. Use frozen foods within the times indicated on page 261 for best results.

COOKING FOOD TO A SAFE TEMPERATURE

Follow these general guidelines to be sure you cook food to an internal temperature that is high enough to kill harmful bacteria. By using a food thermometer to check the temperature of meat, poultry, and other foods, you can ensure that the food is safe to eat and avoid overcooking.

BEEF, VEAL, AND LAMB ROASTS	145°F
BEEF, VEAL, LAMB, GROUND	160°F
PORK	145°F
CHICKEN, TURKEY (whole, pieces, and ground)	165°F
FISH	145°F

STORING LEFTOVERS

To safely store leftovers in your refrigerator, transfer food to clean, shallow covered containers and refrigerate or freeze within 2 hours from cooking time to prevent harmful bacteria from multiplying. Be sure your refrigerator keeps items at 40°F or below. Use these time limits to be sure you do not eat home-refrigerated leftovers that have spoiled.

COOKED SEAFOOD	3 to 4 days
COOKED POULTRY PIECES OR POULTRY DISHES (plain)	3 to 4 days
COOKED POULTRY PIECES COVERED WITH BROTH OR GRAVY	1 to 2 days
COOKED CHICKEN NUGGETS OR PATTIES	1 to 2 days
COOKED MEAT AND MEAT DISHES	3 to 4 days
GRAVY AND MEAT BROTH	1 to 2 days

For more information about storing and cooking foods safely, go to www.foodsafety.gov.

APPENDIX D: **emergency substitutions**

If your recipe calls for	Use
ALLSPICE, 1 teaspoon	½ teaspoon ground cinnamon + 1 teaspoon ground cloves
BAKING POWDER, 1 teaspoon	¼ teaspoon baking soda + ¾ teaspoon cream of tartar
BROWN SUGAR, 1 cup	1 cup granulated sugar + 2 tablespoons molasses
BUTTERMILK, 1 cup	1 tablespoon vinegar or lemon juice + enough fat-free milk to equal 1 cup; or 1 cup fat-free plain yogurt
CAKE FLOUR, 1 cup sifted	1 cup minus 2 tablespoons sifted all-purpose flour
CONFECTIONERS' SUGAR, 1 cup	½ cup plus 1 tablespoon granulated sugar
CORNSTARCH, 1 tablespoon	2 tablespoons all-purpose flour
CRACKER CRUMBS, ¾ cup	¾ to 1 cup plain dry bread crumbs
FLOUR FOR THICKENING, 2 tablespoons all-purpose	1 tablespoon cornstarch
FLOUR, WHOLE-WHEAT (FOR BAKING), 1 cup	$^7/_8$ cup all-purpose flour
FRESH HERBS, 1 tablespoon	1 teaspoon dried herbs
GINGERROOT, PEELED AND GRATED, 1 tablespoon	$^1/_8$ teaspoon ground ginger
HONEY, 1 tablespoon	1 tablespoon plus 1 teaspoon granulated sugar + 1½ teaspoons water
LEMON JUICE, 1 teaspoon	½ teaspoon vinegar
LEMON ZEST, 1 teaspoon	½ teaspoon lemon extract
ONION, 1 small	1 teaspoon onion powder or 1 tablespoon minced dried onion
RICOTTA CHEESE, ½ cup fat-free	½ cup fat-free cottage cheese
SHERRY, 2 tablespoons	1 to 2 teaspoons vanilla extract

If your recipe calls for	Use
SOUR CREAM, 1 cup fat-free	1 cup fat-free plain yogurt
TOMATO JUICE, 1 cup	½ cup no-salt-added tomato sauce + ½ cup water
TOMATO SAUCE, 2 cups	¾ cup no-salt-added tomato paste + 1 cup water
WINE, RED, ½ cup	½ cup fat-free, no-salt-added beef broth or 1 tablespoon balsamic vinegar
WINE, WHITE, ½ cup	½ cup fat-free, low-sodium chicken broth
YEAST, ACTIVE DRY, ¼-ounce package	⅔ ounce cake yeast, crumbled

APPENDIX E: **ingredient equivalents**

Ingredient	Measurement
ALMONDS	1 ounce = ¼ cup slivers
APPLE	1 medium = ¾ to 1 cup chopped; 1 cup sliced
BASIL, fresh	⅔ ounce = ¼ cup leaves, chopped
BELL PEPPER, any color	1 medium = 1 cup chopped or sliced
CARROT	1 medium = ⅓ to ½ cup chopped or sliced; ½ cup shredded
CELERY	1 medium rib = ½ cup chopped or sliced
CHEESE, HARD, such as Parmesan	3½ ounces = 1 cup shredded; 4 ounces = 1 cup grated
CHEESE, SEMIHARD, such as Cheddar, mozzarella, or Swiss	4 ounces = 1 cup grated
CHEESE, SOFT, such as blue, feta, or goat	1 ounce = ¼ cup crumbled
CUCUMBER	1 medium = 1 cup sliced
LEMON JUICE	1 medium = 2 to 3 tablespoons
LEMON ZEST	1 medium = 2 to 3 teaspoons
LIME JUICE	1 medium = 1½ to 2 tablespoons
LIME ZEST	1 medium = 1 teaspoon grated
MUSHROOMS (button)	1 pound = 5 to 6 cups sliced or chopped
ONIONS, GREEN	8 to 9 medium = 1 cup sliced (green and white parts)
ONIONS, white or yellow	1 large = 1 cup chopped; 1 medium = ½ to ⅔ cup chopped; 1 small = ⅓ cup chopped
ORANGE JUICE	1 medium = ⅓ to ½ cup
ORANGE ZEST	1 medium = 1½ to 2 tablespoons grated
STRAWBERRIES	1 pint = 2 cups sliced or chopped
TOMATOES	2 large, 3 medium, or 4 small = 1½ to 2 cups chopped
WALNUTS	1 ounce = ¼ cup chopped

APPENDIX F: **choosing heart-healthy habits**

Your daily habits are powerful contributors to your well-being. Eating a heart-healthy diet as outlined in this book, making physical activity part of your regular routine, maintaining an appropriate weight for your height, not smoking, and not drinking too much alcohol—these are the core essentials of a lifestyle that fosters a healthy body.

Part of taking care of yourself is knowing how your individual health situation affects your risk of developing heart disease and stroke. Work with your healthcare provider and learn about the factors that increase your personal risk. Some, such as advancing age and family history, can't be changed, but many can. You can make the choice to quit smoking, for example. You can work toward losing weight if you need to. Even physical conditions such as high blood pressure, high blood cholesterol, and diabetes can be managed or reduced with a combination of dietary changes, exercise, and medication if recommended. For more information on how to assess your personal risk and develop lasting heart-healthy habits, visit mylifecheck.heart.org.

Be Physically Active. Regular exercise can help you be more physically fit, improve your cardiovascular function, reach and maintain a healthy weight, and boost your confidence. In fact, being physically active offers so many health benefits that the American Heart Association recommends that adults get at least 150 minutes (2 hours and 30 minutes) of moderate-intensity, or 75 minutes (1 hour and 15 minutes) of vigorous-intensity, aerobic physical activity each week. Moderate intensity means that you are able to talk during exercise but not sing. Vigorous activities significantly increase your heart rate, and you should not be able to say more than a few words without having to catch your breath when exercising at this level.

Even a small change in your activity level can improve your health as long as you make that change part of a regular routine. Once you get started, continue to add gradually to reach your target exercise goal. You can accumulate aerobic activity in episodes lasting at least 10 minutes each, preferably spread out through the week. You can also combine moderate and vigorous activities to suit your schedule and preferences to reach an equivalent total.

Reach and Maintain a Healthy Weight. Carrying around extra body weight is not good for your heart in lots of ways. So many Americans can be classified as either overweight or obese that the problem has taken on epidemic proportions. Being overweight is associated with chronic health complications such as high blood pressure, diabetes, and heart disease, to name just a few.

The basic rule of thumb to avoid gaining weight is to use up at least as many calories as you take in. To find out whether you are successfully balancing the calories you eat with how many you burn, visit mylifecheck.heart.org. The information on weight management will show you how to calculate the number of calories you need to maintain your weight. It also discusses how to develop a personal plan to balance the amount and intensity of your physical activity with the number of calories you take in. (The right number of calories to eat each day varies based on your age, gender, and physical activity level and whether you're trying to gain, lose, or maintain your weight.) Making even small changes to keep your weight under control, or lose weight if needed, can add up to a big difference in your long-term health.

Stop Smoking and Moderate Your Use of Alcohol. Smoking increases blood pressure, decreases your ability to exercise, and increases your risk of heart disease, stroke, and cancers. If you currently are a smoker or are regularly exposed to secondhand smoke, find a way to quit or to lessen your exposure. As soon as you get smoking out of your life, your risk of developing health problems begins to drop dramatically.

If you drink alcohol, drink in moderation. That means one drink per day if you're a woman and two drinks per day if you're a man. (One drink equals about 12 ounces of beer, 4 ounces of wine, or 1.5 ounces of hard liquor.) Although there have been reports of some health benefit from moderate use of wine, drinking has a number of downsides, including increased risk of alcoholism, high blood pressure, obesity, stroke, and accidents. Given these and other risks, if you do not already drink alcohol, there is no reason to start.

index